Contemporary Diagnosis and Management of **The Metabolic Syndrome**®

Scott M. Grundy, MD, PhD

Director,
Center for Human Nutrition, and
Chairman,
Department of Clinical Nutrition,
University of Texas Southwestern
Medical Center, Dallas

First Edition

Published by
Handbooks in Health Care Co.,
Newtown, Pennsylvania, USA

Acknowledgment

Ricker Polsdorfer, MD, contributed to the research and writing of this book.

International Standard Book Number: 1-931981-22-1

Library of Congress Catalog Card Number: 2005920825

Table of Contents

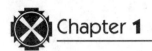

Chapter 1

What Is the Metabolic Syndrome?

Since the middle of the 20th century, steady progress has been made in understanding the fundamental causes of atherosclerotic cardiovascular disease (ASCVD). Population studies, foremost being the Framingham Heart Study, have identified multiple factors associated with increased risk for ASCVD, such as advancing age, insulin resistance, abdominal obesity, cigarette smoking, hypertension, and high serum cholesterol (especially elevated triglycerides and low high-density lipoprotein [HDL] cholesterol). These are called *major risk factors*, and they have been shown to be direct causes of atherosclerotic disease. Studies have also determined the amount of risk inherent in each predisposing condition. Increasing evidence shows that these risk factors are conditioned by genetic and hormonal influences, as well as by acquired conditions, which can be called *underlying risk factors*. These include family history of premature vascular disease, overweight, sedentary lifestyle, and an atherogenic diet. New risk factors, called *emerging risk factors*, have recently been associated with increased risk for ASCVD. Among these are various lipid abnormalities, such as elevated apolipoprotein B (apo B), and small, low-density lipoprotein (LDL) particles, inflammatory factors such as high levels of C-reactive protein, and prothrombotic factors (elevated plasminogen activator inhibitor-1 [PAI-1] and fibrinogen).

In the past decade, researchers have found increasing evidence that different categories of risk factors cluster in individuals and greatly increase the risk for ASCVD. The Framingham study has developed algorithms for summing up the individual contributions of the major risk factors to predict the likelihood of developing ASCVD in the future. In addition, in patients who are obese and sedentary, several risk factors of metabolic origin can combine to raise the risk for ASCVD. This clustering of metabolic risk factors has been named the *metabolic syndrome*.

Numerous clinical trials have demonstrated that therapeutic reduction of the major risk factors will lower the risk for ASCVD. This discovery has been made possible through the development of drugs to better treat hypertension, cholesterol disorders, and insulin resistance.

There is a close relationship between the metabolic syndrome and diabetes, especially type 2 diabetes, which is the most common form. Patients with the metabolic syndrome usually have insulin resistance, which also is a risk factor for type 2 diabetes. Once hyperglycemia develops in a person with the metabolic syndrome, the risk for ASCVD is doubled.

The Metabolic Syndrome: A Multidimensional Risk Factor for Cardiovascular Disease

Many authorities are seeking a clinical definition of the metabolic syndrome. The suggestions for diagnostic criteria for the metabolic syndrome are reviewed in detail in Chapter 5. Although there are differences of opinion about the metabolic syndrome's exact nature, there is no disagreement about its importance, its pervasiveness, or its components.

The National Cholesterol Education Program (NCEP) Expert Panel on Detection, Evaluation, and Treatment of High Blood Cholesterol in Adults (Adult Treatment Panel III) identified five components of the metabolic syndrome

Table 1-1: Defining Components of the Metabolic Syndrome

- Atherogenic dyslipidemia
  - Elevated apolipoprotein B
  - Elevated triglycerides
  - Increased small LDL particles
  - Low HDL cholesterol
- Raised blood pressure
- Insulin resistance ± glucose intolerance
- Proinflammatory state
- Prothrombotic state

that make it a multidimensional risk factor for cardiovascular disease (Table 1-1). It is important to differentiate between the definition of the metabolic syndrome and the clinical criteria required for diagnosis of the condition, which are also provided in ATP III.

Atherogenic Dyslipidemia

One of the most complex and certainly the most extensively studied components of the metabolic syndrome is lipid abnormalities. A particular aggregation of these abnormalities is typical of the metabolic syndrome and the most common abnormality found in type 2 diabetes; that is, elevated concentrations of triglycerides, the presence of small, dense LDL particles, and a low level of HDL cholesterol. Elevated triglycerides are a marker for atherogenic remnant lipoprotein and often for the metabolic syndrome in general. Smaller LDL particles appear to be more atherogenic than larger ones, and are often associated with an increase in the total number of atherogenic apo B-containing lipoproteins (high apo B). A low HDL-C is typically present in patients with metabolic syndrome and is a likely proatherogenic state. The aggregation of these multiple lipoprotein abnormalities definitely indicates a greater risk for ASCVD than revealed by LDL-C concentrations alone.

Elevated Blood Pressure

Hypertension has long been recognized as a major independent risk factor for ASCVD, and is frequently present in patients with the metabolic syndrome. Only recently, however, has there been progress in identifying a causative link between hypertension and other components of the metabolic syndrome. The key cut point as a risk factor is ≥130/85 mm Hg.

Insulin Resistance/Glucose Intolerance

Insulin resistance has been demonstrated to precede both dyslipidemia and hypertension. Insulin also enhances growth factor activity, an effect that could lead to vascular hypertrophy and increased peripheral resistance.[1,2] In addition, both insulin and leptin directly increase sympathetic activity, thereby promoting vasconstriction. Insulin resistance is also a precursor to hyperglycemia.[3]

Insulin resistance is not a simple entity to measure in a clinical setting, but its presence was suspected early in patients with type 2 diabetes because of the coexistence of hyperinsulinemia with hyperglycemia, and a reduced response by many patients with diabetes to exogenous insulin. When researchers developed a technique known as the insulin clamp, they became able to measure insulin resistance quantitatively.[4] In this technique, a patient receives intravenous infusions of insulin and glucose at rates adjusted so that plasma levels remain constant. Determinations of the relative need for insulin and glucose indicate the degree of insulin sensitivity. Insulin clamp studies have identified many features of insulin resistance and its association with components of the metabolic syndrome.

Because glucose clamp studies are impractical for clinical practice, the degree of insulin resistance cannot routinely be measured. However, several factors strongly suggest the presence of increased insulin resistance in a patient: abdominal obesity, impaired fasting glucose (IFG) or impaired glucose tolerance (IGT), and fasting hyperinsulinemia (if insulin measurements are available).

Prothrombotic and Proinflammatory States

A proinflammatory state is characterized by high levels of circulating cytokines, such as tumor necrosis factor-α (TNF-α) and interleukin-6 (IL-6), which is reflected clinically by elevated C-reactive protein (CRP). A prothrombotic state is associated with many thrombotic factors, including fibrinogen, plasminogen activators, antithrombin, von Willebrand factor, factor V Leiden, protein C, and antithrombin. Increased serum CRP and thrombotic markers are associated with increased risk for ASCVD.[5-8]

Secondary Associations

People who have the metabolic syndrome also are prone to an increasing array of secondary conditions (Table 1-2). Much current research is addressing the mechanisms underlying these secondary conditions.

Fatty Liver

Nonalcoholic fatty liver disease (NAFL or NAFLD) is similar to alcoholic fatty liver and was originally mistaken for it. But when it became evident that the metabolic abnormalities related to insulin resistance can also enhance triglyceride accumulation in hepatocytes, NAFL became recognized as among the most common causes of hepatic disease. NAFL has two appearances: a simple, fatty infiltration of hepatocytes, and a more serious steatohepatitis (NASH), which is fatty liver with histologic evidence of both inflammation and fibrosis. Steatohepatitis can sometimes progress to cirrhosis. The conditions appear to represent a failure of the liver to adapt to overwhelming metabolic imbalances, particularly to an increased influx of fatty acids into the liver.[9]

Individuals with obesity and insulin resistance typically have high circulating levels of nonesterified fatty acids (NEFAs), which are derived from lipolysis of triglyceride in adipose tissue. Obesity is accompanied by increased

Table 1-2: Secondary Associations of the Metabolic Syndrome

- Fatty liver
- Polycystic ovary syndrome
- Cholesterol gallstones
- Asthma
- Sleep disturbances
- Sex hormone responsive and colorectal cancer
- Degenerative joint disease
- Hyperuricemia
- Depression
- Albuminuria
- Alzheimer's disease

secretion of NEFA into the circulation. In the presence of insulin resistance in muscle, NEFA uptake is impaired and excess NEFA is diverted to the liver. Both conditions promote NEFA influx into the liver, where fatty acid esterification accumulates hepatic triglyceride. It is also possible that some of the excess fat in liver associated with insulin resistance and its concomitant hyperinsulinemia is caused by increased lipogenesis. In laboratory animals, high insulin levels stimulate lipogenesis in liver.[10]

An unresolved question is why NAFL is transformed into NASH in some patients. Some investigators postulate that excess fatty acids in the liver generate production of cytokines locally, which could lead to hepatic inflammation. Another proposed mechanism is oxidative stress, caused by reactive oxygen species (ROS)—free radicals—in greater abundance than the liver's intrinsic antioxidant capacity can handle. ROS appear to be generated by several mechanisms, the predominant one being a simple mass effect from excess free fatty acid peroxidation.[11] Another is mitochondrial dysfunction, which is worsened by the same oxidative stress to which it contributes. Macrophages, neutrophils, and Kupffer cells also produce ROS.[11]

NAFL has additional causes unrelated (so far) to the metabolic syndrome, including total parenteral nutrition and more than a dozen toxic and pharmacologic agents.

Polycystic Ovary Syndrome

Polycystic ovary syndrome (PCOS) occurs in up to 6% of women in their reproductive years. It has been suggested that PCOS arises from a genetically determined hypersecretion of androgens that encourages preferential abdominal ('android') adiposity, a predecessor of insulin resistance.[12] Another theory holds that genetic forms of insulin resistance underlie PCOS. PCOS coexists with other features of the metabolic syndrome in many women. Obesity either predisposes to PCOS or worsens it. Women with PCOS appear to be at increased risk for both ASCVD and type 2 diabetes.[13]

Cholesterol Gallstones

Cholesterol gallstones occur most often in obese persons, particularly in women and in some ethnic groups (eg, Hispanics and Native Americans). Obesity is accompanied by increased synthesis of cholesterol and formation of bile that is supersaturated with cholesterol.[14] The mechanistic connection between cholesterol gallstones and metabolic syndrome is not entirely clear. However, gallstones often are associated with hyperinsulinemia.[15] Also, Pima Indians with type 2 diabetes[16] have an increased biliary cholesterol saturation index.

Asthma

Little is known of the relationship between metabolic syndrome and asthma, except the fact that it exists.[17] Obesity appears to be a common factor. The increased frequency of asthma in inner city children has been correlated with the increasing prevalence of obesity in this population.[18]

Sleep Disturbances

Obstructive sleep apnea (OSA), also known as sleep disordered breathing (SDB), is a known risk factor for ASCVD, primarily through hypertension from the repetitive stress of hypopnea and the consequent elevation of circulating catecholamines. OSA has demonstrated an association with alterations in sympathovagal balance, baroreceptor sensitivity, and insulin resistance, as well as leptin, growth hormone, and lipid levels.[19] OSA is statistically associated with insulin resistance in obese and nonobese patients.[20]

Some Forms of Cancer

Hormone-sensitive cancers, such as prostate cancer,[21] breast cancer,[22] endometrial cancer,[23] and colorectal cancer,[24] are statistically associated with insulin resistance and the metabolic syndrome. The mechanisms underlying this relationship are poorly understood.

Degenerative Joint Disease

From a mechanical point of view, obesity ravages weight-bearing structures such as the back and knees over time. As more is learned about the pathophysiology of degenerative joint disease, abnormalities in connective tissue, cartilage structure, and synovial fluid may be related to the metabolic changes present in the metabolic syndrome.[25-27]

Hyperuricemia

Numerous studies have found a relationship between hyperuricemia and components of the metabolic syndrome.[28] Multiple statistical correlations make it difficult to determine cause and effect relationships, which will have to come from investigations into the metabolic processes involved.[29,30] Evidence suggests that insulin decreases renal uric acid and sodium clearance.[31-33]

Depression

The association between depression and the metabolic syndrome may be explained by the abnormal increase of stress-related chemical messengers.[34] Depression is associated with polycystic ovary syndrome, which is strongly associated with the metabolic syndrome.[35]

Albuminuria

In patients with noninsulin-dependent diabetes, hyperinsulinemia selectively increases urinary albumin excretion. However, in healthy subjects, insulin has little or no effect on renal hemodynamics, glomerular filtration rate, or permeability to albumin.[32] In a recent Japanese study,[36] insulin resistance, defined as elevated fasting insulin levels, preceded albuminuria and hypertension. The World Health Organization lists microalbuminuria as one of the qualifying criteria of the metabolic syndrome.[37,38]

Alzheimer's Disease

Researchers have recently discovered an apparent association among hyperinsulinemia, diabetes, and Alzheimer's disease (AD). A series of mouse studies from Brigham and Women's Hospital in Boston has identified an enzyme that degrades both insulin and the amyloid β-protein of AD. Researchers hypothesize that excess insulin may consume this enzyme, making too little available for suppressing the accumulation of brain amyloid. On the other hand, a defect in this enzyme may cause both AD and type 2 diabetes, as it did in the subject mice.[39]

Summary

Along with the defining components of the metabolic syndrome—atherogenic dyslipidemia, insulin resistance, elevated blood pressure, prothrombotic states, and proinflammatory states—numerous other diseases and conditions demonstrate a relationship with the metabolic syndrome. The degree of interrelated complexity among all these elements is considerable. Because inflammatory and thrombotic tendencies are part of this syndrome, many more diseases could eventually reside under the expanding umbrella of what we define as the metabolic syndrome. The clinical outcome of foremost significance is ASCVD, and the risk for ASCVD is greatly increased when patients are diagnosed with the metabolic syndrome.

References

1. Third Report of the National Cholesterol Education Program (NCEP) Expert Panel on Detection, Evaluation, and Treatment of High Blood Cholesterol in Adults (Adult Treatment Panel III) final report. *Circulation* 2002;106:3143-3421.

2. Bloomgarden ZT: Obesity, hypertension, and insulin resistance. *Diabetes Care* 2002;25:2088-2097.

3. Palumbo PJ: Gycemic control, mealtime glucose excursions, and diabetic complications in type 2 diabetes mellitus. *Mayo Clin Proc* 2001;76:609-618.

4. DeFronzo RA, Tobin JD, Andres R: Glucose clamp technique: a method for quantifying insulin secretion and resistance. *Am J Physiol* 1979;237:E214-E223.

5. Ridker PM, Morrow DA: C-reactive protein, inflammation, and coronary risk. *Cardiol Clin* 2003;21:315-325.

6. Juhan-Vague I, Alessi MC, Mavri A, et al: Plasminogen activator inhibitor-1, inflammation, obesity, insulin resistance and vascular risk. *J Thromb Haemost* 2003;1:1575-1579.

7. Tracy RP: Inflammation, the metabolic syndrome and cardiovascular risk. *Int J Clin Pract Suppl* 2003;134:10-17.

8. Linton MF, Fazio S: Macrophages, inflammation, and atherosclerosis. *Int J Obes Relat Metab Disord* 2003;27(suppl 3): S35-S40.

9. Mulhall BP, Ong JP, Younossi ZM: Non-alcoholic fatty liver disease: an overview. *J Gastroenterol Hepatol* 2002;17:1136-1143.

10. Day CP: Pathogenesis of steatohepatitis. *Best Pract Res Clin Gastroenterol* 2002;16:663-678.

11. Haque M, Sanyal AJ: The metabolic abnormalities associated with non-alcoholic fatty liver disease. *Best Pract Res Clin Gastroenterol* 2002;16:709-731.

12. Abbott DH, Dumesic DA, Franks S: Developmental origin of polycystic ovary syndrome—a hypothesis. *Endocrinol* 2002;174:1-5.

13. Ovalle F, Azziz R: Insulin resistance, polycystic ovary syndrome, and type 2 diabetes mellitus. *Fertil Steril* 2002;77:1095-1105.

14. Grundy SM, Metzger AL, Adler RD: Mechanisms of lithogenic bile formation in American Indian women with cholesterol gallstones. *J Clin Invest* 1972;51:3026-3043.

15. Misciagna G, Guerra V, Di Leo A, et al: Insulin and gall stones: a population case control study in southern Italy. *Gut* 2000;47:144-147.

16. Bennion LJ, Grundy SM: Effects of diabetes mellitus on cholesterol metabolism in man. *N Engl J Med* 1977;296:1365-1371.

17. O'Brien PE, Dixon JB: The extent of the problem of obesity. *Am J Surg* 2002;184:4S-8S.

18. Rodriguez MA, Winkleby MA, Ahn D, et al: Identification of population subgroups of children and adolescents with high asthma prevalence: findings from the Third National Health and Nutrition Examination Survey. *Arch Pediatr Adolesc Med* 2002; 156:269-275.

19. Coughlin S, Calverley P, Wilding J: Sleep disordered breathing—a new component of syndrome X? *Obes Rev* 2001;2:267-274.

20. Ip MS, Lam B, Ng MM, et al: Obstructive sleep apnea is independently associated with insulin resistance. *Am J Respir Crit Care Med* 2002;165:670-676.

21. Barnard RJ, Aronson WJ, Tymchuk CN, et al: Prostate cancer: another aspect of the insulin-resistance syndrome? *Obes Rev* 2002;3:303-308.

22. Sinagra D, Amato C, Scarpilta AM, et al: Metabolic syndrome and breast cancer risk. *Eur Rev Med Pharmacol Sci* 2002;6:55-59.

23. Hu FB: Overweight and obesity in women: health risks and consequences. *J Womens Health (Larchmt)* 2003;12:163-172.

24. Colangelo LA, Gapstur SM, Gann PH, et al: Colorectal cancer mortality and factors related to the insulin resistance syndrome. *Cancer Epidemiol Biomarkers Prev* 2002;11:385-391.

25. Goldring MB: Osteoarthritis and cartilage: the role of cytokines. *Curr Rheumatol Rep* 2000;2:459-465.

26. Hamerman D, Klagsbrun M: Osteoarthritis. Emerging evidence for cell interactions in the breakdown and remodeling of cartilage. *Am J Med* 1985;78:495-499.

27. van der Kraan PM, van den Berg WB: Anabolic and destructive mediators in osteoarthritis. *Curr Opin Clin Nutr Metab Care* 2000;3:205-211.

28. Vuorinen-Markkola H, Yki-Jarvinen H: Hyperuricemia and insulin resistance. *J Clin Endocrinol Metab* 1994;78:25-29.

29. Rathmann W, Funkhouser E, Dyer AR, et al: Relations of hyperuricemia with the various components of the insulin resistance syndrome in young black and white adults: the CARDIA study. Coronary Artery Risk Development in Young Adults. *Ann Epidemiol* 1998;8:250-261.

30. Clausen JO, Borch-Johnsen K, Ibsen H, et al: Analysis of the relationship between fasting serum uric acid and the insulin sensitivity index in a population-based sample of 380 young healthy Caucasians. *Eur J Endocrinol* 1998;138:63-69.

31. Reaven GM: The kidney: an unwilling accomplice in syndrome X. *Am J Kidney Dis* 1997;30:928-931.

32. Quinones-Galvan A, Ferrannini E: Renal effects of insulin in man. *J Nephrol* 1997;10:188-191.

33. Ter Maaten JC, Voorburg A, Heine RJ, et al: Renal handling of urate and sodium during acute physiological hyperinsulinaemia in healthy subjects. *Clin Sci (Lond)* 1997;92:51-58.

34. Wolkowitz OM, Epel ES, Reus VI: Stress hormone-related psychopathology: pathophysiological and treatment implications. *World J Biol Psychiatry* 2001;2:115-143.

35. Rasgon NL, Rao RC, Hwang S, et al: Depression in women with polycystic ovary syndrome: clinical and biochemical correlates. *J Affect Disord* 2003;74:299-304.

36. Fujikawa R, Okubo M, Egusa G, et al: Insulin resistance precedes the appearance of albuminuria in non-diabetic subjects: 6 years follow up study. *Diabetes Res Clin Pract* 2001;53:99-106.

37. World Health Consultation: Definition, diagnosis, and classification of diabetes mellitus and its complications. Report of the World Health Consultation. Geneva, Switzerland, World Health Organization, 1999.

38. Vega GL: Cardiovascular outcomes for obesity and metabolic syndrome. *Obesity Res* 2002;10(suppl 1):27S-32S.

39. Farris W, Mansourian S, Chang Y, et al: Insulin-degrading enzyme regulates the levels of insulin, amyloid beta-protein, and the beta-amyloid precursor protein intracellular domain in vivo. *Proc Natl Acad Sci U S A* 2003;100:4162-4167.

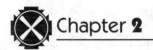 Chapter **2**

Pathogenesis of the Metabolic Syndrome: Underlying Risk Factors

The metabolic syndrome consists of a clustering of metabolic disorders. While each of these disorders independently raises the risk for cardiovascular disease (CVD), the fact that they often occur together suggests that they have common underlying causes. One of the major unresolved issues about the metabolic syndrome is the nature of the underlying causes. This question of underlying cause has generated a major debate in metabolic medicine. One view holds that obesity represents the primary underlying cause of the metabolic syndrome. Another is that an insulin resistance lies at the heart of the syndrome. This chapter and the next will examine the possibility that obesity and insulin resistance are roughly coequal partners underlying the metabolic syndrome.

Obesity and Related Disorders of Adipose Tissue

One of the central features of the metabolic syndrome is the accumulation of excess lipids in critical organs, especially muscle and liver. Lipid accumulation appears to be a driving force behind the development of the metabolic syndrome. Whenever a person is in positive food-energy balance, unused lipids tend to accumulate in various organs.

The role of adipose tissue is to limit this excess accumulation. Adipose tissue serves as a reservoir for excess lipids, reducing the lipid burden on other tissues. As long as adipose tissue performs its function, other tissues are spared the adverse consequences of lipid overload.

Adipose Tissue and Fatty Acid Metabolism
Origins of Adipose Tissue Fat

As a protector against tissue overload, adipose tissue has the capacity to adapt to excess energy input. It can do this in two ways. First, the cells of adipose tissue, adipocytes, can take on more lipids and become enlarged. Second, they can increase in number. Researchers believe that a large number of pre-adipocytes exist and can mature into lipid-laden cells. Moreover, energy overload appears to lead to enhanced adipogenesis, that is, to the formation of new adipocytes.

Of the two major sources of nutrient fuel—fat and carbohydrate—only fat can be stored in large quantities. Some excess carbohydrate can be stored in the form of glycogen, but not much. Instead, excess carbohydrate is largely converted into fat for storage in adipose tissue. Excess fat is likewise stored in adipose tissue. Fat is stored in the form of triglyceride, which consists of three molecules of fatty acid bound to glycerol, hence 'triglyceride.' Lipids enter and leave adipose tissue in the form of nonesterified fatty acids (NEFA). Fatty acids are esterified into triglycerides in adipocytes, as they are stored.

Fatty acids can reach adipose tissue from two sources. First, dietary fat has a direct route to adipose tissue through chylomicrons. These consist of triglyceride-rich lipoproteins (TGRLP) that are formed in the intestine from dietary fat. Chylomicrons enter the circulation through the thoracic duct and pass into capillaries. An enzyme on the endothelial surface of capillaries, lipoprotein lipase (LPL), hydrolyzes the triglycerides into fatty acids. The capillaries in adipose tissue beds are particularly rich in LPL;

hence most of newly released fatty acids are able to enter adipose tissue directly. Lesser amounts of fatty acids pass into the systemic circulation as NEFA and are removed by other tissues.

A second source of adipose tissue lipid comes from very low-density lipoproteins (VLDL), which are formed in the liver. The triglyceride of VLDL also undergoes lipolysis by LPL, and the resulting fatty acids also enter adipose tissue.

Regulation of Adipose Tissue Lipolysis

A primary function of adipose tissue is to store nutrient energy for the body during fasting. The mobilization of energy in the form of NEFA is highly regulated. The key enzyme for lipolysis of triglycerides into glycerol and NEFA is hormone-sensitive lipase (HSL). This enzyme is activated through cyclic AMP-dependent phosphokinase (PKA). It is well known that β-adrenergic agents increase cyclic AMP, activating PKA to phosphorylate HSL. Another key protein in the lipolytic process is perilipin. This protein surrounds the lipid droplet, and it, too, must be phosphorylated for lipolysis to proceed. Perilipin apparently delays lipolysis by blocking access of HSL to fat droplets. Upon phosphorylation, perilipin allows HSL to contact the triglyceride and to begin lipolysis. Rates of lipolysis of adipose triglyceride are highly sensitive to circulating insulin concentrations. High plasma insulin suppresses phosphorylation of HSL and perilipin, which inhibits lipolysis and NEFA release. Thus, in the postprandial state, when insulin levels are high, plasma NEFA concentrations are low. Conversely, during fasting, when plasma insulin falls, NEFA concentrations rise.

In obese persons, fasting plasma NEFA is elevated compared to nonobese subjects. During feeding, NEFA concentrations fall, but often not to the levels observed in the nonobese. Thus, adipose tissue seems to be 'insulin resistant' to lipolysis in obese persons. The explanation for adipose-tissue insulin resistance is not fully understood, but several possibilities can be considered. First, the adipocytes are enlarged from engorgement with large fat droplets. Consequently, amounts of perilipin surrounding these droplets may be insufficient to block access of HSL. As a result, rates of lipolysis may be greater than normal in the fasting state. Moreover, in most obese individuals, the number of adipocytes is increased. Thus, if each adipocyte has a basal rate of lipolysis, even in the fasting state, total lipolysis will be greater than normal. For both of these reasons, obese persons will have elevated plasma NEFA concentrations.

Excess NEFA and Insulin Resistance in Muscle

The major site of NEFA use is skeletal muscle. Most of the NEFA entering muscle is oxidized and used for energy. However, considerable evidence indicates that excess NEFA entering muscle interferes with muscle uptake of glucose. Interruption of insulin-mediated glucose disposal in muscle is the classic definition of insulin resistance. The inverse of insulin resistance is insulin sensitivity. The latter can be measured in the whole body by the glucose-clamp technique, by adjusting plasma levels of glucose and insulin through intravenous injection to achieve steady-state concentrations of each. From rates of infusion, it is possible to estimate rates of insulin-mediated glucose disposal, or insulin sensitivity. Other methods have been introduced to estimate insulin sensitivity, including a modified glucose-clamp technique (minimal model), glucose and insulin responses to oral glucose challenges, fasting insulin levels, and equations with fasting glucose and insulin levels (HOMA insulin resistance). Most authorities consider these other methods inferior to the glucose-clamp technique, but in truth they all measure something slightly different. Therefore, the definition of insulin sensitivity is to a large extent method-dependent. But all methods show that, on average, obese persons have a reduced insulin sensitivity compared to nonobese persons (ie, they are more insulin resistant).

To understand how excess NEFA causes insulin resistance we must review the basic mechanisms of insulin action. These mechanisms are outlined in Figure 2-1.

Insulin is the principal anabolic hormone in the body. It is a major cytokine, participating in multiple gene expression and signal transduction pathways, by which it increases cell membrane importation of glucose, regulates substrate availability to the Krebs cycle and intracellular protein and lipid pathways, and increases glycogen storage, protein synthesis, and lipogenesis, while inhibiting glycogenolysis, glycolysis, gluconeogenesis, lipolysis, and protein breakdown. Many other metabolic effects of insulin have been identified.

The mechanisms by which high plasma NEFA reduces insulin sensitivity are not fully understood. This observation was first made by Randle et al[1] in the early 1960s. Subsequently, Randle proposed the existence of a glucose-fatty acid cycle in which fatty acids suppress oxidation of glucose.[2] According to the Randle hypothesis, fatty acid oxidation will lead to accumulation of acetyl-CoA, which will inhibit pyruvate dehydrogenase (PDH), causing accumulation of citrate. Citrate, in turn, will inhibit phosphofructokinase (PFK), leading to accumulation of glucose-6-phosphate (G6P) and decreasing hexokinase (HK) activity. Consequently, glucose uptake by muscle cells will be decreased. Conversely, the hypothesis implies that increases in carbohydrate oxidation should decrease fatty acid oxidation. Some evidence supports this mechanism. Although the Randle hypothesis held sway for many years, its mechanistic proof has remained elusive. Alternate mechanisms have been proposed whereby fatty acid accumulation may cause insulin resistance in muscle.

According to another hypothesis, excess fatty acids in muscle cells cause insulin resistance by activation of a serine kinase cascade. Serine phosphorylation results in reduced tyrosine phosphorylation of insulin-stimulated insulin receptor substrate (IRS)-1, which in turn reduces IRS-

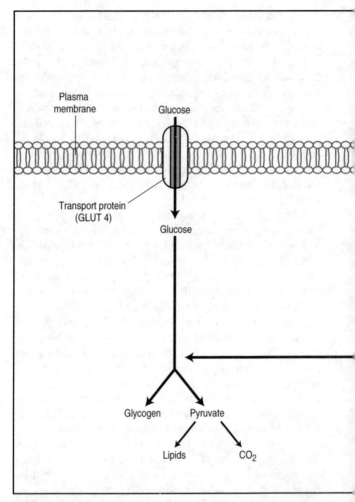

Figure 2-1: Insulin pathways. Insulin is the principal anabolic hormone in the body. It is a major cytokine, participating in multiple gene expression and signal transduction pathways, by which it increases cell membrane importation of glucose, regulates substrate availability to

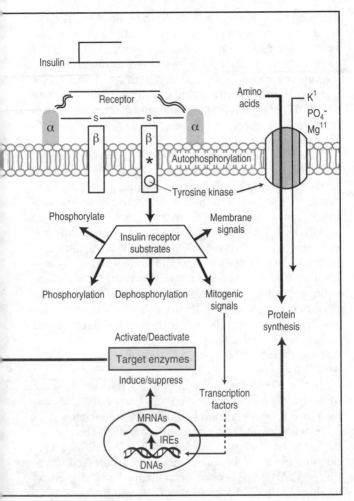

the Krebs cycle and intracellular protein and lipid pathways, and increases glycogen storage, protein synthesis and lipogenesis while inhibiting glycogenolysis, glycolysis, gluconeogenesis, lipolysis, and protein breakdown.[1] Many metabolic effects of insulin have been identified.

1-linked phosphatidylinositol 3-kinase activity. The latter is a required step in insulin-stimulated glucose transport into muscle with glucose transporter 4 (GLUT4).[3] How fatty acids activate serine kinase is under investigation. One theory is that increased influx of NEFA into muscle increases intracellular fatty acetyl-CoA and diacylglycerol (DAG) concentrations. Increased DAG then activates protein kinase C-θ (PKC-θ), which increases serine-phosphorylated IRS-1.[4]

Besides increased input of NEFA in muscle, factors that modify fatty acid metabolism in muscle also could lead to greater intracellular concentrations of fatty acids and DAG, setting into motion the above changes. Another regulatory system that may be implicated involves malonyl-CoA. For example, activation of PKC isoforms could increase malonyl-CoA, which will block fatty acid oxidation and increase intracellular fatty acid-CoA levels, which in turn can exacerbate down-regulation of insulin signaling.[5] Although these pathways become exceedingly complex, they illustrate that insulin resistance associated with high NEFA level is multifactorial and incompletely understood.

Excess NEFA, Atherogenic Dyslipidemia, and Fatty Liver

When NEFA levels are high in obese persons, some of the excess NEFA enters the liver. Liver fatty acids can have two fates. A portion is oxidized in mitochondria to carbon dioxide and water or to ketone bodies. The remainder is reesterified and incorporated into VLDL for secretion into plasma. Obese persons have an increased secretion of VLDL triglyceride[6,7] accompanied by an increased production of VLDL-apo B and LDL-apo B.[8,9]

Obesity further leads to increased activity of hepatic lipase observed in obese persons.[10,11] Hepatic lipase is an enzyme that is expressed on the surface of liver cells. When its activity is high, high-density lipoprotein (HDL) particles are degraded. Small HDL particles are characteristic of atherogenic dyslipidemia, as are low HDL-C concentrations.

When the influx of fatty acids into liver is excessive, triglycerides usually accumulate in the liver. The result, fatty liver, is becoming increasingly common in the United States.[12] In some persons, fatty liver is associated with inflammation. Fatty liver plus hepatic inflammation is known as nonalcoholic steatohepatitis (NASH). Occasionally, the inflammation progresses to fibrosis, or cirrhosis of the liver.

Adipose Tissue as a Source of Inflammatory Cytokines

Adipose tissue can produce and secrete cytokines (eg, tumor necrosis factor-α [TNF-α] and interleukins [IL], particularly IL-1β and IL-6). These cytokines appear to have a biologic function within adipose tissue and possibly in systemic tissue. Within adipose tissue, they appear to stimulate lipolysis and to promote fatty acid mobilization. They also may modulate the functional characteristics of adipocytes.[13] In systemic tissues, adipose tissue-derived cytokines may enhance insulin resistance. The hypothesized mechanism for the latter is through serine phosphorylation of IRS-1, which blocks insulin signaling.[14]

A marker for increased cytokine activity is the release of C-reactive protein (CRP), an acute-phase reactant that is produced in the liver. Obese individuals have higher levels of serum CRP than do thin persons.[15]

Role of Leptin in the Metabolic Syndrome

Leptin is a hormone that is released by adipocytes. Its primary function is to regulate food intake. Leptin was discovered from studies of ob/ob mice, which lack functional leptin,[16] have voracious appetites, and exhibit an obesity syndrome. Leptin interacts with leptin receptors in the brain. The hormone likely plays an important role in energy homeostasis through regulation of eating behavior and sympathetic nervous system modulation. In addition, there has been considerable interest in the possibility that leptin has a direct peripheral action, thereby affecting metabolism in muscle, liver, and pancreas. Increased amounts of leptin are released in obese persons. Some evidence supports the concept that leptin promotes β-oxidation of fatty acids, thereby reducing insulin resistance.[17] Because obese persons secrete large amounts of leptin and yet accumulate fat in various tissues, a state of leptin resistance has been proposed, but its role as a cause of insulin resistance and the metabolic syndrome remains to be determined.

Coagulation and Fibrinolysis Abnormalities in Obesity

Obese persons are at increased risk from venous and arterial thrombotic events. Obesity is associated with increased plasma concentrations of prothrombotic factors such as fibrinogen, von Willebrand factor (vWF), factor VII, and plasminogen activator inhibitor-1 (PAI-1).[18] Particularly well established is an increase in circulating PAI-1 in obesity. PAI-1 is the major inhibitor of plasminogen activation. Adipose tissue makes several substances that can up-regulate PAI-1, including transforming growth factor β, TNF-α, angiotensin II, and interleukin 6.[19] The stromal cells of adipose tissue appear to be mainly responsible for production of PAI-1.[20] The various abnormalities in coagulation and fibrinolysis associated with obesity appear to underlie the prothrombotic state of the metabolic syndrome.

Adiponectin and Insulin Resistance

Another adipokine implicated in the development of the metabolic syndrome is adiponectin.[21] In some animal models, a fall in expression of adiponectin is accompanied by insulin resistance. Conversely, increases in adiponectin increase insulin sensitivity. One of its mechanisms may be a reduction in secretion of NEFA by adipose tissue. When adiponectin levels are low, triglyceride levels increase in muscle and liver and reduce insulin resistance. A low expression of adiponectin may be secondary to the local release of inflammatory cytokines by the liver.

Body Fat Distribution and the Metabolic Syndrome

Patterns of Fat Distribution

Body fat can accumulate in several different adipose tissue compartments. Most fat accumulates in subcutaneous adipose tissue, while smaller amounts are located within the abdomen. Intra-abdominal fat can accumulate in either the intraperitoneal compartment or the retroperitoneal region. Intraperitoneal fat also is called visceral fat.

Subcutaneous fat typically is divided into lower body and upper body fat. Lower body fat is mainly in the gluteofemoral region, while most upper body subcutaneous fat is in the trunk. Two general patterns of obesity are recognized: predominant upper body obesity and predominant lower body obesity. Upper body obesity is characterized by fat located in truncal subcutaneous and visceral compartments. Typically, about two thirds of truncal fat is subcutaneous, with the remainder being visceral. However, the ratio of truncal subcutaneous fat to visceral fat varies. Some persons have disproportionate amounts of visceral fat. When this occurs, the person is said to have visceral obesity. But in those people who have visceral obesity, most of the fat is still subcutaneous. Another name for upper body fat is abdominal obesity. This term is used because an increase in abdominal girth is the most easily recognized feature of fat deposited predominantly in the trunk.

In the clinical setting, two parameters related to body fat are recognized: body mass index (BMI) and waist circumference. The BMI is calculated as kilograms of body weight divided by height in meters squared (kg/m^2). The BMI is positively correlated with total body fat. It is not the best measure of total body fat, but it can be easily used in routine clinical practice. More accurate measures of total body fat can be obtained by underwater weighing,[22] bioelectrical impedance,[23,24] and total body potassium.[25] Bioelectrical impedance measurements make use of a simple instrument that records surface electrical potentials. Because these various methods typically are not available in physicians' offices, the BMI is an acceptable surrogate for total body fat. According to current guidelines in the United States, BMI measurements correlating with overweight and obesity are as follows:

Weight Category	BMI (kg/m^2)
Normal	20-24.9
Overweight	25-29.9
Obesity	>30

The obesity category can also be divided into class I, II, and III, with BMIs of 30-34.9, 35-39.9, and >40, respectively. The specific category of abdominal obesity is defined as follows:

Gender	Waist circumference
Men	>40 inches (>102 cm)
Women	>35 inches (>88 cm)

For reasons not fully understood, abdominal obesity is more strongly correlated with the risk factors of the metabolic syndrome than is BMI. In particular, people who have upper body obesity are more likely to exhibit the metabolic syndrome than those with lower body obesity. For the population as a whole, obese men typically manifest upper body obesity (android obesity), while obese women usually have lower body obesity (gynoid obesity). However, some women show upper body obesity, and some men have lower body obesity. Also, among those with upper body obesity, some have more severe forms in which almost all fat is present in the trunk.

Some populations appear to be particularly sensitive to excess adipose tissue and will develop the metabolic syndrome with lesser degrees of obesity. This is particularly true in several Asian populations. For this reason, the cut points for both obesity and abdominal obesity are being reassessed in various populations, and obesity cut points are becoming increasingly country-specific.

Causes of Upper Body Obesity
Sex Hormones

Because men typically develop upper body obesity while women are prone to lower body obesity, hormonal factors could explain different patterns of fat distribution. In support, upper body obesity occurs in women with polycystic ovarian syndrome (PCOS), who have been shown to be in a state of hyperandrogenemia. They also develop the metabolic syndrome more often than do women with lower body obesity. Despite this strong circumstantial evidence, it has not been demonstrated with certainty that excess androgens are responsible for most cases of upper body obesity. Other mechanisms have been implicated.

Hypercorticoidism

Patients subject to excess corticosteroids—those with Cushing's disease or therapy with exogenous corticosteroids—develop an abnormal pattern of fat distribution that resembles upper body obesity. Body fat is redistributed to the upper body, making the 'buffalo hump' of corticosteroid excess well recognized. Some investigators[26] have postulated that upper body obesity is the result of excessive corticosteroid action, either from high circulating levels of corticosteroids or from increased intracellular sensitivity to corticosteroid stimulation.

Genetic Susceptibility

Some ethnic groups appear to be genetically susceptible to upper body obesity. Most prominent among these groups are South Asians. Abdominal obesity is the major feature when many South Asians become even mildly overweight. South Asians carry increased susceptibility for the metabolic syndrome and type 2 diabetes.

Other populations also have a relatively high frequency of predominantly upper body obesity, such as the Hispanic population, which is also diabetes prone. Among American whites, upper body obesity is much less common than in South Asians and Hispanics, but when present, it is accompanied by increased risk for diabetes and the metabolic syndrome.

Primary Insulin Resistance
as a Cause of Upper Body Obesity

Although many commonly believe that upper body obesity is a cause of insulin resistance, another possibility is that primary insulin resistance causes accumulation of fat in the upper body. If insulin resistance in adipose tissue causes increased lipolysis, it could deplete fat stores in gluteofemoral fat. Even if there is a slight difference in propensity for uptake or release of fatty acids from one fat compartment vs another, then over time, one compartment could accumulate more fat than another. This could be the result of a metabolic disturbance such as primary insulin resistance. This potential mechanism remains to be thoroughly evaluated. If it applies, a rethinking of the relationship between upper body obesity and insulin resistance may be required.

Lower Body Fat Deficiency

If endocrine or genetic factors were to produce a deficiency of lower body adipose tissue, upper body obesity might develop by default. Factors determining rates of adipogenesis in different body compartments are not understood. For example, androgens might suppress adipogenesis in the gluteofemoral region, while estrogens might promote it. Regulators of adipogenesis have come under intense investigation. Differential regulation in different adipose compartments could potentially modify primary sites of fat accumulation.

Upper Body Obesity vs Lower Body Obesity

Most investigators agree that persons with upper body obesity are more susceptible to the metabolic syndrome than are those with lower body obesity. The mechanisms for these differences are not fully understood, but persons with upper body obesity have higher plasma levels and turnover rates of NEFA.[27] These higher levels could induce insulin resistance in skeletal muscle and cause lipid overload in the liver. Also, upper body adipose tissue may release more proinflammatory and prothrombotic factors than lower body adipose tissue. The difference in propensity for the metabolic syndrome between upper and lower body obesities is generally well accepted. Opinion differs, however, on the contribution of different adipose tissue compartments in the upper body.

Upper Body Obesity:
Subcutaneous Fat vs Visceral Fat

Differences in opinion also exist between the relative importance of visceral obesity and subcutaneous obesity. Both sides present impressive arguments. For example, excess adipose tissue in the intraperitoneal space releases large amounts of NEFA directly into the portal vein, which leads directly to the liver. If this mechanism dominates, then changes in the liver itself could be mainly responsible for the metabolic syndrome. Overloading the liver with fat will contribute to atherogenic dyslipidemia and promote gluconeogenesis and increased hepatic glucose output, which in turn should enhance peripheral insulin resistance. Recent studies, moreover, suggest that visceral adipose tissue is a rich source of inflammatory cytokines and PAI-1, both of which could exacerbate the metabolic syndrome.

On the other hand, excess subcutaneous adipose tissue carries the potential for detrimental effects as well. Because the mass of adipose tissue in the subcutaneous compartment of the trunk is typically two to three times that of intraperitoneal fat, total release of NEFA from this compartment should exceed that of intraperitoneal fat. Abate et al[28] demonstrated that abdominal subcutaneous fat is more highly correlated with insulin resistance than is visceral fat. Moreover, Jensen et al[29] report that most of the excess NEFA entering the circulation comes from subcutaneous adipose tissue. In fact, of the total amount of NEFA entering the liver, more is derived from subcutaneous adipose tissue than from visceral adipose tissue.[29] This fact weakens the argument that visceral adipose tissue is all-important in determining the metabolic complications of upper body obesity.

Whole Body Obesity

Besides the well-known difference in typical adipose tissue deposition between women and men, women are more likely to exhibit truncal subcutaneous obesity than visceral obesity. If waist circumference is taken as a measure of upper body obesity, many women will have both abdominal obesity and gluteofemoral obesity. In other words, when obesity in women becomes more severe, they will exhibit whole body obesity. However, the upper body component of their obesity is characterized largely by truncal subcutaneous obesity. They will have much less visceral obesity than will men with comparable amounts of body fat accumulation. Limited data suggest that women with upper body obesity will have as much peripheral insulin resistance as comparable men. Women also manifest a similar prevalence of type 2 diabetes. In contrast, men, who have more visceral obesity than women, are more likely to exhibit atherogenic dyslipidemia.

Role of Primary Insulin Resistance

Obesity in its different forms is an insulin-resistant state. Obese adipose tissue can be considered to be insulin resistant because fasting plasma levels of NEFA are elevated even in the face of fasting hyperinsulinemia. In skeletal muscle, insulin-mediated glucose disposal is typically reduced in obese patients. It is commonly believed that the metabolic syndrome is 'caused' by insulin resistance. But there is strong evidence that obesity causes insulin resistance. Furthermore, as stated before, obesity can influence the development of metabolic risk factors unrelated to obesity. Therefore, we might ask whether insulin resistance occurring independently of obesity might cause the metabolic syndrome.

What Is Primary Insulin Resistance?

Insulin resistance can occur independently of obesity. We can define primary insulin resistance as a genetic defect in the insulin-signaling pathway that gives rise to insulin resistance. Figure 2-1 summarizes the complex pathways of insulin signaling that could be defective in syndromes of primary insulin resistance. Insulin action begins by insulin binding to the insulin receptor. When the alpha and beta subunits of the receptor interact, they catalyze tyrosine kinase activity. This activity initiates a cascade of phosphorylation/dephosphorylation reactions that are responsible for the downstream actions of insulin.[30] Insulin receptor substrates-1 and -2 (IRS-1 and IRS-2) appear to be the primary targets of the insulin receptor tyrosine kinase. IRS-1 and IRS-2 undergo tyrosine phosphorylation at several locations on the molecules for activation. IRS-1 mediates the insulin signal through subsequent interaction with signaling molecules containing Src homology 2 domains.[31] Phosphorylation of IRS-1 activates a number of serine/threonine protein kinases, which, through cascades, elicit multiple intracellular reactions. The result is a complex of signaling networks. The actions of insulin are not the same in every tissue and depend on key intracellular effectors.[32]

One of the targets of insulin action is the lipid kinase phosphatidylinositide 3-kinase (PI-3 kinase), which facilitates glucose uptake into cells. Glucose entry into the cell is mediated by glycosylated membrane proteins named glucose transporters (GLUTs). Several GLUTs with different tissue specificity have been identified: GLUT 1 (most tissues), GLUT 2 (liver, pancreatic β-cells), GLUT 3 (brain), and GLUT 4 (skeletal muscle, heart, adipocytes). Besides affecting glucose transport, insulin regulates glucose and lipid metabolism at several sites via downstream cascades. In some cases, insulin action increases protein activity through phosphorylation. In others, it inhibits protein function by phosphorylation. It can also regulate enzyme activity by increasing or decreasing formation of molecules that act as allosteric modifiers. Finally, insulin's downstream products can directly modify gene action by acting on promoter regions of DNA.

Primary Forms of Insulin Resistance
Mutations and Polymorphisms
in Insulin Signaling Pathway

Rare patients are homozygous for mutations in insulin receptor genes that give rise to autosomal recessive disorders and severe insulin resistance.[33] Examples include leprechaunism and Rabson-Mendenhall syndrome. The former is the more severe: infants with leprechaunism show growth restriction, abnormal glucose metabolism, and, usually, death before 1 year of age. Rabson-Mendenhall syndrome is less severe. Affected persons usually live to be to 5 to 15 years of age. These rare abnormalities seemingly do not cause the metabolic syndrome.

Other postreceptor proteins contain reported polymorphisms that may cause insulin resistance, which in turn predisposes to metabolic syndrome or type 2 diabetes. Known polymorphisms occur in IRS-1[34-36] and IRS-2.[37,38] Ongoing investigations are attempting to confirm the metabolic significance of these polymorphisms.

Another type of gene polymorphism that appears to affect insulin signaling occurs in the large, class II exoprotein, protein PC-1. Overexpression of PC-1 in cultured cells impairs insulin receptor tyrosine kinase activity and other cellular responses to insulin.[39] Studies in human populations have demonstrated a positive association between a polymorphism in PC-1 and insulin resistance.[40,41] Abate et al[42] showed that this polymorphism is strongly associated with insulin resistance in South Asians, in whom insulin resistance is common. Overexpression or abnormal expression of PC-1 may interfere with insulin binding to its receptor.

Polygenic Forms of Primary Insulin Resistance

Beyond rare mutations and polymorphisms in insulin signaling, increased insulin resistance is enriched in certain ethnic groups. This increased prevalence of primary insulin resistance presumably has a polygenic basis. Examples include South Asians and, among whites, offspring of diabetic parents. In the white population, insulin sensitivity varies somewhat independently of obesity. This variability may be caused in part by genetic differences in the efficacy of insulin signaling pathways.

The population of the Indian subcontinent has a high prevalence of both type 2 diabetes and coronary heart disease. Particularly susceptible are South Asians who migrate to Western countries. They are unusually insulin resistant.[43-46] It has been uncertain whether insulin resistance in migrant Asians is primary or secondary to abdominal obesity. A high prevalence of diabetes was detected in urban populations in India itself.[47] Recent studies from our laboratory have demonstrated that South Asians are insulin resistant independent of abdominal obesity.[48-50] This finding strongly suggests that insulin resistance in South Indians is genetic, possibly related to defective insulin signaling. The close association between a polymorphism for PC-1 and insulin resistance in South Asians supports this concept.[42]

Young adult whites who have two diabetic parents have a high prevalence of primary insulin resistance.[51-53] Genetic defects in insulin signaling have not been identified, but the likelihood is high. Finally, in the general white population, occurrence of insulin resistance is often independent of obesity, which again suggests a genetic contribution.[54,55] Thus, primary insulin resistance almost certainly exists and contributes to the metabolic syndrome. At the same time, it is likely that when persons are genetically susceptible to insulin resistance, the coexistence of obesity plays a key role in eliciting the metabolic syndrome.

Acquired Insulin Resistance Independent of Obesity

Insulin Resistance of Aging

Insulin resistance increases with age. Aging commonly leads to a change in body composition characterized by a higher percentage of body fat and loss of skeletal muscle.[56] These changes likely enhance insulin resistance. Some recent evidence, however, suggests that aging itself can impair insulin signaling independent of changes in body composition.[57] For example, many older men have acquired mitochondrial defects in oxidation of fatty acids in skeletal muscle.[58] These defects apparently impair insulin sensitivity. Finally, some investigators speculate that insulin resistance is secondary to an increasing proinflammatory state with aging.[59,60]

Physical Inactivity

Increasing physical activity reduces insulin resistance.[61-64] Exercise exerts a direct effect on skeletal muscle to promote glucose uptake.[65] It acts through a variety of mechanisms.[66,67] Because exercise reduces insulin resistance, sedentary life habits presumably will enhance insulin resistance. Certainly regular physical activity reduces metabolic risk factors.

Autoimmune Insulin Resistance

Protease Inhibitors

Long-term treatment of HIV with protease inhibitors causes lipodystrophy in many patients. Changes in body composition alone redistribute body fat to skeletal muscle and liver and could lead to development of insulin resistance. Moreover, protease inhibitors can acutely induce insulin resistance.[68-70] The mechanism for this effect is not known, but speculation centers on impairment of translocation of GLUT 4 transporters to the surface of skeletal muscle cells.

Summary

This chapter examines the pathogenesis of the metabolic syndrome, from its potential origins in either obesity and related disorders of adipose tissue or in insulin resistance. Both obesity and insulin resistance play significant roles. The following chapter continues the discussion of pathogenesis by examining the origins of individual components of the metabolic syndrome—atherogenic dyslipidemia, hypertension, impaired insulin secretion, and prothrombotic and proinflammatory states.

References

1. Randle PJ, Garland PB, Hales CN, et al: The glucose fatty-acid cycle. Its role in insulin sensitivity and the metabolic disturbances of diabetes mellitus. *Lancet* 1963;1:785-789.

2. Randle PJ: Regulatory interactions between lipids and carbohydrates: the glucose fatty acid cycle after 35 years. *Diabetes Metab Rev* 1998;14:263-283.

3. Petersen KF, Shulman GI: Pathogenesis of skeletal muscle insulin resistance in type 2 diabetes mellitus. *Am J Cardiol* 2002;90: 11G-18G.

4. Yu C, Chen Y, Cline GW, et al: Mechanism by which fatty acids inhibit insulin activation of insulin receptor substrate-1 (IRS-1)-associated phosphatidylinositol 3-kinase activity in muscle. *J Biol Chem* 2002;277:50230-50236.

5. Ruderman NB, Saha AK, Vavvas D, et al: Malonyl-CoA, fuel sensing, and insulin resistance. *Am J Physiol* 1999;276:E1-E18.

6. Grundy SM, Mok HY, Zech L, et al: Transport of very low density lipoprotein triglycerides in varying degrees of obesity and hypertriglyceridemia. *J Clin Invest* 1979;63:1274-1283.

7. Egusa G, Beltz WF, Grundy SM, et al: Influence of obesity on the metabolism of apolipoprotein B in humans. *J Clin Invest* 1985; 76:596-603.

8. Kesaniemi YA, Grundy SM: Increased low density lipoprotein production associated with obesity. *Arteriosclerosis* 1983;3:170-177.

9. Kesaniemi YA, Beltz WF, Grundy SM: Comparisons of metabolism of apolipoprotein B in normal subjects, obese patients, and patients with coronary heart disease. *J Clin Invest* 1985;76:586-595.

10. Nie L, Wang J, Clark LT, et al: Body mass index and hepatic lipase gene (LIPC) polymorphism jointly influence postheparin plasma hepatic lipase activity. *J Lipid Res* 1998;39:1127-1130.

11. Carr MC, Hokanson JE, Zambon A, et al: The contribution of intraabdominal fat to gender differences in hepatic lipase activity and low/high density lipoprotein heterogeneity. *J Clin Endocrinol Metab* 2001;86:2831-2837.

12. Haque M, Sanyal AJ: The metabolic abnormalities associated with non-alcoholic fatty liver disease. *Best Pract Res Clin Gastroenterol* 2002;16:709-731.

13. Coppack SW: Pro-inflammatory cytokines and adipose tissue. *Proc Nutr Soc* 2001;60:349-356.

14. Hotamisligil GS: Mechanisms of TNF-alpha-induced insulin resistance. *Exp Clin Endocrinol Diabetes* 1999;107:119-125.

15. Tchernof A, Nolan A, Sites CK, et al: Weight loss reduces C-reactive protein levels in obese postmenopausal women. *Circulation* 2002;105:564-569.

16. Friedman JM, Halaas JL: Leptin and the regulation of body weight in mammals. *Nature* 1998;395:763-770.

17. Muoio DM, Lynis Dohm G: Peripheral metabolic actions of leptin. *Best Pract Res Clin Endocrinol Metab* 2002;16:653-666.

18. De Pergola G, Pannacciulli N: Coagulation and fibrinolysis abnormalities in obesity. *J Endocrinol Invest* 2002;25:899-904.

19. Mutch NJ, Wilson HM, Booth NA: Plasminogen activator inhibitor-1 and haemostasis in obesity. *Proc Nutr Soc* 2001;60: 341-347.

20. Alessi MC, Morange P, Juhan-Vague I: Fat cell function and fibrinolysis. *Horm Metab Res* 2000;32:504-508.

21. Matsuzawa Y, Funahashi T, Kihara S, et al: Adiponectin and metabolic syndrome. *Arterioscler Thromb Vasc Biol* 2004;24:29-33.

22. Tolli J, Bengtsson BA, Bosaeus I, et al: A comparison of different methods to measure body composition in patients. *Appl Radiat Isot* 1998;49:469-472.

23. Kyle UG, Genton L, Karsegard L, et al: Single prediction equation for bioelectrical impedance analysis in adults aged 20-94 years. *Nutrition* 2001;17:248-253.

24. Bolanowski M, Nilsson BE: Assessment of human body composition using dual-energy x-ray absorptiometry and bioelectrical impedance analysis. *Med Sci Monit* 2001;7:1029-1033.

25. Brodowicz GR, Mansfield RA, McClung MR, et al: Measurement of body composition in the elderly: dual energy x-ray absorptiometry, underwater weighing, bioelectrical impedance analysis, and anthropometry. *Gerontology* 1994;40:332-339.

26. Rivera MP, Svec F: Is cortisol involved in upper-body obesity? *Med Hypotheses* 1989;30:95-100.

27. Jensen MD, Haymond MW, Rizza RA, et al: Influence of body fat distribution on free fatty acid metabolism in obesity. *J Clin Invest* 1989;83:1168-1173.

28. Abate N, Garg A, Peshock RM, et al: Relationships of generalized and regional adiposity to insulin sensitivity in men. *J Clin Invest* 1995;96:88-98.

29. Guo Z, Hensrud DD, Johnson CM, et al: Regional postprandial fatty acid metabolism in different obesity phenotypes. *Diabetes* 1999;48:1586-1592.

30. Kahn CR, Goldfine AB: Molecular determinants of insulin action. *J Diabetes Complications* 1993;7:92-105.

31. White MF: The IRS-1 signaling system. *Curr Opin Genet Dev* 1994;4:47-54.

32. Nystrom FH, Quon MJ: Insulin signalling: metabolic pathways and mechanisms for specificity. *Cell Signal* 1999;11:563-574.

33. Longo N, Wang Y, Smith SA, et al: Genotype-phenotype correlation in inherited severe insulin resistance. *Hum Mol Genet* 2002; 11:1465-1475.

34. Berger D, Barroso I, Soos M, et al: Genetic variants of insulin receptor substrate-1 (IRS-1) in syndromes of severe insulin resistance. Functional analysis of Ala513Pro and Gly1158Glu IRS-1. *Diabet Med* 2002;19:804-809.

35. Marini MA, Frontoni S, Mineo D, et al: The Arg972 variant in insulin receptor substrate-1 is associated with an atherogenic profile in offspring of type 2 diabetic patients. *Clin Endocrinol Metab* 2003;88:3368-3371.

36. Esposito DL, Li Y, Vanni C, et al: A novel T608R missense mutation in insulin receptor substrate-1 identified in a subject with type 2 diabetes impairs metabolic insulin signaling. *J Clin Endocrinol Metab* 2003;88:1468-1475.

37. Stefan N, Kovacs P, Stumvoll M, et al: Metabolic effects of the Gly1057Asp polymorphism in IRS-2 and interactions with obesity. *Diabetes* 2003;52:1544-1550.

38. Lautier C, El Mkadem SA, Renard E, et al: Complex haplotypes of IRS2 gene are associated with severe obesity and reveal heterogeneity in the effect of Gly1057Asp mutation. *Hum Genet* 2003;113:34-43.

39. Goldfine ID, Maddux BA, Youngren JF, et al: Role of PC-1 in the etiology of insulin resistance. *Ann N Y Acad Sci* 1999;892: 204-222.

40. Gu HF, Almgren P, Lindholm E, et al: Association between the human glycoprotein PC-1 gene and elevated glucose and insulin levels in a paired-sibling analysis. *Diabetes* 2000;49:1601-1603.

41. Frittitta L, Baratta R, Spampinato D, et al: The Q121 PC-1 variant and obesity have additive and independent effects in causing insulin resistance. *J Clin Endocrinol Metab* 2001;86:5888-5891.

42. Abate N, Carulli L, Cabo-Chan A Jr, et al: Genetic polymorphism PC-1 K 12 1Q and ethnic susceptibility to insulin resistance. *J Clin Endocrinol Metab* 2003;88:5927-5934.

43. McKeigue PM, Marmot MG, Syndercombe Court YD, et al: Diabetes, hyperinsulinaemia, and coronary risk factors in Bangladeshis in east London. *Br Heart J* 1988;60:390-396.

44. McKeigue PM, Shah B, Marmot MG: Relation of central obesity and insulin resistance with high diabetes prevalence and cardiovascular risk in South Asians. *Lancet* 1991;337:382-386.

45. McKeigue PM, Pierpoint T, Ferrie JE, et al: Relationship of glucose intolerance and hyperinsulinaemia to body fat pattern in south Asians and Europeans. *Diabetologia* 1992;35:785-791.

46. McKeigue PM, Ferrie JE, Pierpoint T, et al: Association of early-onset coronary heart disease in South Asian men with glucose intolerance and hyperinsulinemia. *Circulation* 1993;87:152-161.

47. Singh RB, Niaz MA, Agarwal P, et al: Epidemiologic study of central obesity, insulin resistance and associated disturbances in the urban population of North India. *Acta Cardiol* 1995;50:215-225.

48. Chandalia M, Abate N, Garg A, et al: Relationship between generalized and upper body obesity to insulin resistance in Asian Indian men. *J Clin Endocrinol Metab* 1999;84:2329-2335.

49. Chandalia M, Abate N, Cabo-Chan AV Jr, et al: Hyperhomocysteinemia in Asian Indians living in the United States. *J Clin Endocrinol Metab* 2003;88:1089-1095.

50. Chandalia M, Cabo-Chan AV Jr, Devaraj S, et al: Elevated plasma high-sensitivity C-reactive protein concentrations in Asian Indians living in the United States. *J Clin Endocrinol Metab* 2003; 88:3773-3776.

51. Frayling TM, Walker M, McCarthy MI, et al: Parent-offspring trios: a resource to facilitate the identification of type 2 diabetes genes. *Diabetes* 1999;48:2475-2479.

52. Carlsson M, Wessman Y, Almgren P, et al: High levels of nonesterified fatty acids are associated with increased familial risk of cardiovascular disease. *Arterioscler Thromb Vasc Biol* 2000;20:1588-1594.

53. Straczkowski M, Kowalska I, Stepien A, et al: Insulin resistance in the first-degree relatives of persons with type 2 diabetes. *Med Sci Monit* 2003;9:CR186-190.

54.   Jones CN, Abbasi F, Carantoni M, et al: Roles of insulin resistance and obesity in regulation of plasma insulin concentrations. *Am J Physiol Endocrinol Metab* 2000;278:E501-E508.

55.   McLaughlin T, Abbasi F, Lamendola C, et al: Differentiation between obesity and insulin resistance in the association with C-reactive protein. *Circulation* 2002;106:2908-2912.

56.   Basu R, Breda E, Oberg AL, et al: Mechanisms of the age-associated deterioration in glucose tolerance: contribution of alterations in insulin secretion, action, and clearance. *Diabetes* 2003;52: 1738-1748.

57.   Clevenger CM, Parker Jones P, Tanaka H, et al: Decline in insulin action with age in endurance-trained humans. *J Appl Physiol* 2002;93:2105-2111.

58.   Petersen KF, Befroy D, Dufour S, et al: Mitochondrial dysfunction in the elderly: possible role in insulin resistance. *Science* 2003;300:1140-1142.

59.   Roubenoff R: Catabolism of aging: is it an inflammatory process? *Curr Opin Clin Nutr Metab Care* 2003;6:295-299.

60.   Bruunsgaard H: Effects of tumor necrosis factor-alpha and interleukin-6 in elderly populations. *Eur Cytokine Netw* 2002;13:389-391.

61.   Segal KR, Edano A, Abalos A, et al: Effect of exercise training on insulin sensitivity and glucose metabolism in lean, obese, and diabetic men. *J Appl Physiol* 1991;71:2402-2411.

62.   Perseghin G, Price TB, Petersen KF, et al: Increased glucose transport-phosphorylation and muscle glycogen synthesis after exercise training in insulin-resistant subjects. *N Engl J Med* 1996; 335:1357-1362.

63.   Houmard JA, Tanner CJ, Slentz CA, et al: The effect of the volume and intensity of exercise training on insulin sensitivity. *J Appl Physiol* 2004;96:101-106.

64.   Reynolds TH 4th, Brown MD, Supiano MA, et al: Aerobic exercise training improves insulin sensitivity independent of plasma tumor necrosis factor-alpha levels in older female hypertensives. *Metabolism* 2002;51:1402-1406.

65.   Goodyear LJ, Kahn BB: Exercise, glucose transport, and insulin sensitivity. *Annu Rev Med* 1998;49:235-261.

66.   Koval JA, Maezono K, Patti ME, et al: Effects of exercise and insulin on insulin signaling proteins in human skeletal muscle. *Med Sci Sports Exerc* 1999;31:998-1004.

67. Borghouts LB, Keizer HA: Exercise and insulin sensitivity: a review. *Int J Sports Med* 2000;21:1-12.

68. Noor MA, Seneviratne T, Aweeka FT, et al: Indinavir acutely inhibits insulin-stimulated glucose disposal in humans: a randomized, placebo-controlled study. *AIDS* 2002;16:F1-F8.

69. Woerle HJ, Mariuz PR, Meyer C, et al: Mechanisms for the deterioration in glucose tolerance associated with HIV protease inhibitor regimens. *Diabetes* 2003;52:918-925.

70. Koster JC, Remedi MS, Qiu H, et al: HIV protease inhibitors acutely impair glucose-stimulated insulin release. *Diabetes* 2003;52:1695-1700.

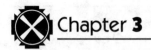

Chapter 3

Pathogenesis of the Metabolic Risk Factors

The metabolic risk factors for the metabolic syndrome include atherogenic dyslipidemia, elevated blood pressure, elevated glucose level (or glucose intolerance), a prothrombotic state, and a proinflammatory state. Underlying risk factors (obesity and related disorders of adipose tissue and insulin resistance) contribute to the development of these factors. Each metabolic risk factor can also be worsened by specific abnormalities unrelated to underlying risk factors.

Atherogenic Dyslipidemia

Atherogenic dyslipidemia consists of elevated serum triglyceride-rich lipoproteins (TGRLP), elevated total apolipoprotein B (apo B; non-high-density lipoprotein [HDL] cholesterol), small low-density lipoprotein (LDL) particles, and low HDL (Table 3-1). It is influenced by underlying risk factors and by dysregulation of other, specific factors. The cause of each abnormality of atherogenic dyslipidemia will be reviewed first.

Elevated Very Low-Density Lipoprotein Triglycerides and Apo B
Underlying Risk Factors

Obesity contributes to overproduction of very low-density lipoprotein (VLDL) triglycerides and VLDL apolipoprotein B (apo B).[1-3] The increased influx of non-

**Table 3-1: Factors Associated
With Development of
Atherogenic Dyslipidemia**

Underlying risk factors:

Obesity and related disorders of adipose tissue

Insulin resistance

Low-fat, high-carbohydrate diets

Specific abnormalities:

Elevated VLDL triglyceride total apolipoprotein B

Defective oxidation of fatty acids

Defective catabolism of triglyceride-rich lipoproteins

Lipoprotein lipase deficiency (extremely rare)

Apolipoprotein CII deficiency (extremely rare)

High serum levels and polymorphisms of
apolipoprotein CIII

Apolipoprotein E2 genotype

Apolipoprotein A5 polymorphisms

Defective LDL receptor-mediated clearance of
apolipoprotein B-containing lipoproteins

esterified fatty acids (NEFA) into the liver in obesity causes hepatic overload of lipid. Excess lipid in the liver promotes the formation of VLDL particles, causing overproduction of VLDL triglyceride and VLDL apo B. Whether primary insulin resistance, independent of obesity, causes the same changes is uncertain. Nonetheless, when adipose tissue is insulin resistant, NEFA release is high.

Various dietary factors beyond obesity also raise VLDL production. High intakes of alcohol and carbohydrates en-

Specific Abnormalities (continued):

Low HDL-cholesterol

>Elevated serum triglyceride levels

>Increased activity of hepatic lipase

>Increased activity of cholesterol ester transport protein (CETP)

>Reduced synthesis of apolipoprotein A1

>Genetic abnormalities in ABC A1 transporters

Small LDL particles

>Elevated triglyceride levels

>Overproduction of apo-B containing lipoproteins

VLDL = very low-density lipoprotein, LDL = low-density lipoprotein, HDL = high-density lipoprotein

hance hepatic secretion of VLDL triglyceride but apparently do not increase secretion of VLDL apo B. The reasons for this dissociation are unclear.

Specific Abnormalities

Fatty acid oxidation defects

When obesity and/or insulin resistance drive surplus NEFA into the liver, these fatty acids can either be oxidized or re-esterified and incorporated into VLDL triglycerides. Fatty acid oxidation requires several key enzymes, some of which may be genetically defective.[4] Rare genetic disorders of fatty acid oxidation are accompanied by hypertriglyceridemia.[5]

Defective catabolism of triglyceride-rich lipoproteins

Many specific defects in the catabolism of TGRLP result in higher levels of serum triglyceride and remnant lipoproteins. The most severe is an inherited deficiency of lipoprotein lipase (LPL), an enzyme required for lipolysis of triglyceride in VLDL and chylomicrons. Rare individuals are homozygous for mutations in this enzyme and are unable to catabolize TGRLP. Consequently, they develop severe hypertriglyceridemia. Although these homozygous mutations are rare, many polymorphisms in LPL have been identified[6] that in the heterozygous state cause minor rises in serum triglyceride concentrations. When they occur in obese persons, triglyceride levels can rise substantially, causing atherogenic dyslipidemia. Other polymorphisms in LPL will likely be identified in the future.

Another apolipoprotein, apo CII, is required for lipolysis of TGRLP. It activates LPL. Rare patients lack apo CII and thus manifest severe hypertriglyceridemia.[7] Moderate reductions in apo CII are innocuous; only small amounts are required to activate LPL. A sister apolipoprotein involved in lipolysis of VLDL triglyceride is apo CIII. This apolipoprotein, in contrast to apo CII, inhibits LPL. These two apolipoproteins may act in concert to modulate TGRLP lipolysis. Polymorphisms in the promoter region of apo CIII exist. These polymorphisms apparently enhance expression of apo CIII and increase the amount present on VLDL particles. High levels of apo CIII can override the action of apo CII and thereby raise triglyceride levels.[8] Furthermore, high apo CIII interferes with the interaction of VLDL remnants with LDL receptors, causing higher remnant levels. Subgroup analysis of lipid-lowering clinical trials suggests that high levels of apo CIII-containing remnants promote coronary atherogenesis.[9]

Another class of apolipoproteins affecting VLDL metabolism is the apo E's. Three isoforms of apo E occur: E4, E3, and E2. These isoforms can result in six genotypes: E4:E4; E4:E3; E4:E2; E3:E3; E3:E2, and E2:E2. The E4:E4 genotype is accompanied by relatively high LDL-cholesterol levels; it also associates with premature Alzheimer's disease. The E2:E2 genotype produces a defect in interaction of VLDL remnants with LDL receptors, thereby raising remnant concentrations. These remnants contain large amounts of cholesterol esters and are called β-VLDL. When E2:E2 occurs in association with overproduction of VLDL, severe remnant accumulation ensues.[10] This condition, *familial dysbetalipoproteinemia*, represents one form of atherogenic dyslipidemia.

Apolipoprotein A5 was discovered so recently that its function is not yet known, but one polymorphism in this protein is accompanied by higher triglyceride levels.[11] Thus, it could be one of several proteins that influence the development of atherogenic dyslipidemia in persons who are predisposed to the disorder by either obesity or primary insulin resistance.

Elevated apo-B-containing lipoproteins caused by defective LDL receptors

The LDL receptors remove LDL from the circulation. Defects in the LDL receptors lead to elevations of LDL levels.[12] LDL receptors additionally remove VLDL remnants; hence, they lower all apo B-containing lipoproteins. Expression of LDL receptors varies greatly. Dietary and genetic factors regulate LDL-receptor synthesis. In particular, high intakes of dietary saturated fats and cholesterol suppress the synthesis of LDL receptors.[13] Although polymorphisms in LDL receptors may modify expression, the synthesis of these receptors appears to be related more to polymorphisms in factors regulating receptor expression than to those in the LDL receptor itself. Although

LDL receptor activity is related primarily to concentrations of LDL, it also affects VLDL remnant concentrations. Low expression of LDL receptors thus raises total apo B concentrations, which is one of the components of atherogenic dyslipidemia.

Low HDL-Cholesterol

Underlying Risk Factors

Obesity is accompanied by low HDL-cholesterol levels.[14] Multiple mechanisms may be responsible: elevated triglyceride levels, increased activity of hepatic lipase, increased activity of cholesterol-ester transfer protein (CETP), and even a higher plasma volume for dilution of HDL particles.[15] Many persons with low HDL levels are also insulin resistant. High intakes of carbohydrate (low-fat diets) can reduce HDL concentrations.

Specific Abnormalities

Elevated triglyceride

When triglycerides are elevated, HDL-cholesterol levels decrease because triglyceride in TGRLP exchanges with HDL cholesterol ester.

Increased activity of hepatic lipase

This enzyme is located on the surface of hepatocytes. It is a lipase for lipoprotein triglycerides and phospholipids and degrades larger HDL particles into smaller ones. Increases in activity of hepatic lipase reduce levels of HDL cholesterol.

Rare patients have a genetic absence of hepatic lipase.[16] They have increases in HDL cholesterol, triglycerides, and apo A-I. Studies carried out in collaboration with the author have provided new insights into the regulation of hepatic lipase activity, with implications for the metabolic syndrome. These studies and those of other workers have shown that persons who have elevations of hepatic lipase activity typically have features of the metabolic syndrome.[17-19] Conversely, persons with a low activity of hepatic lipase usually have elevated HDL cholesterol concentrations. Investigations of hepatic lipase activities and gene polymorphisms have revealed that African-American men typically have polymorphic patterns that reduce hepatic lipase activities and raise HDL-cholesterol levels.[20] Lower activities of hepatic lipase in African-American men provide one explanation of why this population has a relatively low prevalence of atherogenic dyslipidemia, one of the key features of the metabolic syndrome.

Increased activity of cholesterol ester transfer protein (CETP)

CETP is a circulating protein that transfers cholesterol esters from HDL to VLDL and LDL.[21] High levels of CETP will reduce HDL-cholesterol concentrations. Conversely, low levels of CETP produce higher HDL cholesterol concentrations. Drugs are now under development that inhibit the activity of CETP for the purpose of raising HDL levels. Although CETP activities are known to influence HDL-cholesterol concentrations and lipoprotein composition, it is not known whether CETP plays a significant role in the development of atherogenic dyslipidemia characteristic of the metabolic syndrome.

Reduced synthesis of apolipoprotein A1

Rare disorders result from failure to synthesize apo A-I, the major apolipoprotein of HDL. Little evidence supports the concept that defects in the synthesis of apo A-I contribute significantly to the development of atherogenic dyslipidemia.

Genetic abnormalities in ABC A1 transporters

One of the factors that appears to regulate HDL levels is the adenosine triphosphate-binding cassette protein A1 (ABC A1) transporter. This transporter plays a role in reverse cholesterol transport, ie, in the removal of cholesterol from peripheral tissue and transport to the liver for excretion. Recent work suggests that these transporters play a role in modulating the levels of plasma HDL and in regulating intracellular cholesterol in the liver as well as in peripheral cells.[22] Several mutations or polymorphisms have been identified in ABC A1 transporter that are associated with reduced levels of HDL.[23] Although low HDL levels are a feature of atherogenic dyslipidemia of the metabolic syndrome, it is unclear that dysfunction of ABC A1 transporters plays a role.

Small LDL Particles

When triglyceride concentrations are elevated, LDL particles tend to be smaller and to show greater heterogeneity (polydispersity). Small LDL particles are another lipoprotein abnormality accompanying atherogenic dyslipidemia. The mechanisms for formation of small LDL particles appear to be similar, at least in part, to those of small HDL particles (ie, the exchange of triglyceride in TGRLP with cholesterol ester in LDL.) Additionally, it has been postulated that overproduction of apo B-containing lipoproteins results in a unique form of TGRLP that is destined to become small LDL particles. Regardless of mechanism, small LDL particles as one of the constituents of atherogenic dyslipidemia is commonly found in patients with the metabolic syndrome.

Elevated Blood Pressure

The elevation of blood pressure accompanying the metabolic syndrome is often only moderate. Many persons exhibiting other metabolic risk factors have a high-normal blood pressure level (systolic 130 to 139 mm Hg and/or diastolic 85 to 89 mm Hg). Recently the Seventh Joint National Commission (JNC 7) report[24] introduced a new category of blood pressure called *prehypertension*. This category consists of blood pressure in the range of 120 to 139 mm Hg systolic and 80 to 89 mm Hg diastolic. It was introduced in the belief that most persons with blood pressures in this range will eventually develop categoric hypertension (blood pressure >140/90 mm Hg). Evidence was presented that this prehypertension carries some increased risk for coronary heart disease (CHD) and stroke,

Table 3-2: Mechanisms of Elevated Blood Pressure in Persons With the Metabolic Syndrome

Underlying risk factors:

- Obesity
- Insulin resistance
- Dietary factors
- Aging

Specific abnormalities:

- Increased renal sodium reabsorption
- Enhanced cardiac output secondary to central nervous system hyperactivity
- Peripheral vasoconstriction
  - Neuro-adrenergic mediation
  - Angiotensin mediated
- Glucocorticoids and aldosteronism
- Inflammation
- Specific, multifactorial (polygenic) causation

at least compared to blood pressures in the desirable range. Moreover, JNC 7 postulated that prehypertension is caused mainly by underlying risk factors such as obesity, physical inactivity, and a hypertensive diet. These underlying risk factors of course contribute to higher blood pressures even in patients with categoric hypertension.

This chapter will next explain the role of underlying risk factors and abnormalities specific to blood pressure regulation (Table 3-2). The regulation of blood pressure is as complex as the pathogenesis of hypertension. For this reason, much of any discussion of pathogenesis must fall into the area of speculation. Although there has been much conjecture about a role of genetics in the etiology of hypertension, a clear picture has yet to be developed. Research into the genetics of hypertension nonetheless is active and may provide insights in the future.

Underlying Risk Factors for Hypertension

Obesity

Overweight and obesity contribute significantly to raising blood pressure levels in many populations. For almost any population or subgroup, levels of blood pressure on average are higher in overweight/obese persons than in lean individuals. The mechanisms underlying this association are not well understood, but several factors have been implicated. These include increases in peripheral resistance and increases in blood volume leading to a higher cardiac output. Of the several implicated factors, an increased reabsorption of sodium is highly suspect.[25] Enhanced sodium reabsorption has been attributed to an elevated glomerular filtration rate as well as to increased renal blood flow.[26] Hall et al further speculate that altered intrarenal physical forces secondary to kidney compression by excess adipose tissue are yet another factor increasing sodium reabsorption. This and other mechanisms may be responsible for activation of the renal-angiotensin system, which in turn may impair natriuresis.[27] Increased angiotensin will raise peripheral resistance even further. Moreover, obese persons appear to have an over-active sympathetic nervous system, which will increase cardiac output and raise peripheral resistance. Overproduction of leptin accompanying obesity may raise blood pressure further, possibly through interaction of leptin with other neurochemical pathways in the hypothalamus, including melanocortin-4 receptors.[28] Many of these pathways are at present conjectural, but continue to be foci of ongoing research.

Insulin resistance

Much interest has focused on the possibility that insulin resistance raises blood pressure. Several studies demonstrate that people with hypertension are insulin resistant.[28,29] This fact undoubtedly engendered the concept of a cause-and-effect relationship (ie, insulin resistance causes hypertension). With this focus, it follows that obesity contributes to higher blood pressure through insulin resistance.

Several of the pathways to hypertension once attributed to obesity likewise have been attributed to insulin resistance. Despite interest in the role of insulin resistance in blood pressure elevation, the mechanistic relationship remains undetermined. Moreover, epidemiologic studies indicate that certain populations carrying a high burden of insulin resistance, such as South Asians and Native Americans, are not particularly prone to hypertension. In other words, in the presence of isolated primary insulin resistance, the frequency of hypertension does not appear to be increased. For this reason, insulin resistance per se may not be a major cause of hypertension. This contrasts to the almost certain role of obesity as a cause of high blood pressure, whatever the mechanisms.

Dietary factors

The concept that dietary factors independent of obesity elevate blood pressure has evoked interest in the public health community. Considerable epidemiologic and clinical research has been carried out to test this hypothesis. Several dietary components have been put forward as potential factors in the development of hypertension. These include high intakes of sodium, calcium, and fat, as well as low intakes of potassium, fruits, and vegetables. Considerable data support the concept that some individuals are 'salt sensitive' and undergo a rise in blood pressure with high-salt diets. Up to one third of the population is believed to be susceptible to salt-induced hypertension.

The relationship between high calcium intake and hypertension is less well established. The likelihood that dietary factors are important in the etiology of hypertension has led to experimentation with diets designed to improve nutrient composition as it relates to blood pressure. One widely tested diet is the Dietary Approaches to Stop Hypertension (DASH) diet,[30] which is low in fat and high in fruits, vegetables, and fiber, and tends to be low in sodium and high in potassium. Rigid adherence to the DASH diet causes a moderate reduction in blood pressure in hypertensive patients.

Aging

Blood pressure tends to rise with age. Age-associated increases in systolic blood pressure are common. Multiple mechanisms have been implicated,[31] including stiffening of the large arteries secondary to cross-linking of collagen. A generalized arterial vasoconstriction possibly related to arteriolar thickening might be an additional factor. Some investigators question whether these changes should be linked to the metabolic syndrome, because they have no obvious connection to metabolism. On the other hand, beyond these arterial changes, weight gain with aging is common and thus will elicit obesity-associated causes of hypertension. Even when weight gain does not occur, a loss of muscle mass signifies an increase in percentage of total body fat, which may in itself bring obesity-associated mechanisms into play. These same changes raise insulin resistance, and if the latter contributes to elevated blood pressure, it could contribute to the problem in older persons. Without doubt, changes in body composition can cause metabolic alteration.

Specific Abnormalities

Specific abnormalities in blood pressure regulation may be either genetic or acquired. Several possible abnormalities are listed in Table 3-2, which considers several acquired factors with the underlying risk factors. Studies are now underway to determine whether genetic variation modifies these potential sites of abnormality in a way that raises blood pressure. Of particular interest is whether the interaction of underlying risk factors with specific abnormalities may produce an additive or synergistic rise in blood pressure.

A few monogenic causes of hypertension have been identified. Most notable are glucocorticoid-mediated aldosteronism, mineralocorticoid excess, and Little's disease.[32] Genome scans in families have identified promising regions for novel hypertension genes, including chromosomes 2q, 3p, 14 (around 41cM), and 19.[33-35] Additionally, potentially functional polymorphisms that appear to associate with higher blood pressure have been reported for several genes: 11 β-hydroxysteroid dehydrogenase type 2,[36] adducing,[37] G-protein β3 subunit 825T allele,[38] G protein-coupled receptor kinase (GRK type 4),[39] as well as angiotensinogen (AGT), angiotensin I-converting enzyme (ACE), and angiotensin II type 1 receptor (eg, AT1R +1166 A/C polymorphism).[40] Polymorphisms in Cd36 fatty acid transporter have been implicated in spontaneous hypertension in the rat.[41]

Because no single gene polymorphisms have been identified as major causes for common forms of hypertension, current speculation centers on a probable polygenic causation. Moreover, several acquired factors may be required to interact with a polygenic substrate to elicit clinical hypertension. Thus, the causation of elevated blood pressure accompanying the metabolic syndrome follows a parallel pathogenesis with other metabolic risk factors.

Impaired Insulin Secretion and Hyperglycemia

An elevation of plasma glucose, either in the fasting or postprandial state, is one risk factor for the metabolic syndrome. Clinical criteria identify three categories of hyperglycemia: diabetes mellitus (fasting glucose >126 mg/dL or 2-hour postprandial glucose >200 mg/dL), impaired fasting glucose (IFG) (100 to 125 mg/dL), and impaired glucose tolerance (IGT) (2-hour postprandial glucose >140 mg/dL). Insulin resistance is an underlying risk factor for the development of hyperglycemia. However, as long as pancreatic β-cell function is normal, insulin secretion will be sufficient to maintain normoglycemia even with insulin resistance. Only when β-cell function declines does hyperglycemia develop. The usual progression of plasma glucose deterioration is through three stages: IGT, IFG, and diabetes. Some persons, however, go directly from IGT to diabetes with an undetectably short period of IFG. The form of diabetes that results from a combination of insulin resistance and reduced insulin secretion is called type 2 diabetes.

Factors leading to deterioration of β-cell function leading to type 2 diabetes are not well understood. The pathophysiology of β-cell dysfunction represents one of the greatest unresolved problems in diabetes research. Extensive investigation into this problem has nonetheless uncovered potential mechanisms, which are listed in Table 3-3. They can be divided into loss of β-cells and impairment of β-cell function.

Patients with type 2 diabetes usually maintain considerable reserve in insulin secretory capacity, although it is not sufficient to forestall forever the development of hyperglycemia in the presence of insulin resistance. Several studies suggest that part of the problem, particularly in those with advanced type 2 diabetes, is a reduction in the total number of pancreatic β-cells. Cell death has been reported to be from apoptosis of β-cells,[42] perhaps with depletion of intracellular calcium causing activation of caspase-12.[43] Activation of caspase-12 is a known mechanism for apoptosis. Other investigations suggest that prolonged hyperglycemia will kill β-cells (glucotoxicity), as may prolonged elevation of plasma NEFA (lipotoxicity).[44] Finally, a good case has been made for the killing of β-cells by amyloidosis.[45] If so, this appears to be a relatively late phenomenon in the course of type 2 diabetes. One study showed that severe insulin resistance accompanying generalized lipodystrophy was accompanied by advanced amyloidosis of pancreatic β-cells and type 2 diabetes relatively early in life.[46] The extent to which β-cell

Table 3-3: Pathophysiology of Impaired Insulin Secretion by Pancreatic β-Cells

Loss of β-cells

Apoptosis of β-cells

> Depletion of intracellular Ca2+ stores with subsequent activation of caspase-12

> Glucotoxicity (hyperglycemia) and lipotoxicity (high NEFA levels)

> Amyloidosis of β-cells causing cell death (late phenomenon)

Impaired β-cell function

> - β-Cell exhaustion (prolonged insulin resistance)

> - Decreased β-cell responsiveness to glucose

> - Possible impairment of β-cell glucose oxidation

> Inability of glucose to potentiate other islet nonglucose β-cell secretagogues

> - Signaling abnormalities in the metabolism of malonyl-CoA and long chain CoA

> - Glucotoxicity (hyperglycemia) and lipotoxicity (high NEFA levels)

> - Amyloid fibril impairment of β-cell function (early)

> - Aging of β-cells

NEFA = nonesterified fatty acids

amyloidosis occurs in usual cases of type 2 diabetes, however, is unclear. Current views are that it may be a factor in the decline of β-cell function, although it is unlikely to be the primary or major cause.

Impairment of β-cell function may also explain a deterioration in the ability to produce enough insulin to overcome insulin resistance and to prevent hyperglycemia. Such an impairment could occur without death of β-cells because of structural or functional changes. β-Cells could be exposed to the same aging influences that occur in other tissues, eg, methylation of DNA with loss of function.[47] Moreover, accumulation of amyloid fibrils in β-cells may impair their ability to secrete insulin.[48] Changes of these types may be irreversible and may account for the fact that a progressive and seemingly irreversible decline in β-cell function occurs in persons with type 2 diabetes.

A commonly proposed hypothesis is that β-cells undergo 'exhaustion' secondary to prolonged overstimulation of insulin secretion in the presence of insulin resistance. The nature of this exhaustion is unknown. Because many obese persons with insulin resistance never develop type 2 diabetes, the existence of β-cell exhaustion is questionable. Still, prolonged insulin resistance occurring with other β-cell defects could well accelerate a decline in insulin secretory capacity. It further has been proposed that prolonged hyperglycemia or elevated NEFA levels can induce functional impairment of insulin secretion.[49] In this case, glucotoxicity and lipotoxicity may be reversible and without lasting damage to β-cell structure. Certainly a decreased β-cell responsiveness to glucose has been observed.[49] Additionally, responsiveness is to some extent restorable on reversal of insulin resistance (eg, by weight reduction). One characteristic of decreased β-cell responsiveness is the inability of glucose to potentiate other islet nonglucose β-cell secretagogues.[50] The molecular basis of deterioration in insulin-secretory capacity is unknown. It has, however, been proposed that one mechanism is an impairment of glucose oxidation in β-cells.[51] Another proposal is the possibility of signaling abnormalities in the metabolism of malonyl-CoA or long-chain fatty acid CoAs.[51]

Prothrombotic State

Individuals with the metabolic syndrome typically exhibit elevations of procoagulant factors in the blood. Together, these factors constitute a prothrombotic state. Specific defects in the coagulation system undoubtedly worsen a tendency to arterial thrombosis in many people. Current concepts of the causes of a prothrombotic state are listed in Table 3-4.

The most consistent coagulation defect associated with the metabolic syndrome is an elevation of PAI-1 levels. An important discovery was that adipose tissue can synthesize and secrete PAI-1.[52,53] Recent reports indicate that visceral adipose tissue is particularly capable of producing PAI-1.[54] Accumulation of fat in the liver may be a further stimulus for the hepatic synthesis of PAI-1.[55] Whether insulin resistance unrelated to obesity can produce elevations in PAI-1 remains to be demonstrated with certainty. Nonetheless, evidence supporting an independent action of insulin resistance has been reported.[56-58] The source of high PAI-1 levels because of insulin resistance is unknown. Still, if adipose tissue is insulin resistant, adipocytes may also be the source. Beyond these underlying risk factors, more specific causes of elevations of PAI-1 may be an activation of the renin-angiotensin-aldosterone system (RAAS)[59] or genetic polymorphisms in the PAI-1.[59] If these additional abnormalities are present in a person with the metabolic syndrome, increases in PAI-1 levels could be accentuated.

Elevations of plasma fibrinogen comprise another component of the prothrombotic state and the metabolic syndrome.[60] Several causes of high plasma fibrinogen have been reported (Table 3-4). Cigarette smoking is a well-recognized cause.[61] Other causes more closely related to the metabolic syndrome are obesity[54] and insulin resistance.[62] A likely explanation for the increase in fibrinogen in obesity and insulin resistance is the greater production of inflammatory cytokines.[63] In some patients, the adverse effect of obesity and insulin resistance on fibrino-

Table 3-4: Causes of a Prothrombotic State

- Elevated plasma plasminogen activator inhibitor-1 (PAI-1)
  - Obesity, especially abdominal obesity
  - Fatty liver
  - Insulin resistance
  - Activated renin-angiotensin-aldosterone system
  - Genetic polymorphisms of PAI-1 gene

- Elevated plasma fibrinogen
  - Smoking
  - Obesity
  - Insulin resistance
  - Genetic polymorphisms of fibrinogen
  - Increased cytokine production (inflammation)

- Elevated von Willebrand's factor (vWF)

- Elevated plasma factor VII
  - Increased plasma triglycerides

gen levels may be accentuated by genetic polymorphisms in the fibrinogen gene that enhance the synthetic response to other influences.[64]

Other procoagulant factors have been reported to be present in the prothrombotic state. These include elevations of von Willebrand's factor (vWF), factor VII, tissue plasminogen activator (tPA) antigen (which represents t-PA/PAI-1 complexes that indicate antifibrinolysis), factor V Leiden, protein C, and antithrombin III. Increases in factor VII have been reported to be present in those with hypertriglyceridemia.[65] Similarly, increases in tissue plasminogen activator antigen occur in persons with obesity,[66] insulin resistance,[67] and hypertriglyceridemia.[68]

- Elevated tissue plasminogen activator (tPA)
  antigen (which represents t-PA/PAI-1 complexes
  indicative of antifibrinolysis)
  - Obesity
  - Insulin resistance
  - Hypertriglyceridemia

- Elevated factor V Leiden

- Elevated protein C

- Elevated antithrombin III

- Enhanced platelet activity
  - Smoking
  - Diabetes
  - Obesity and hyperleptinemia
  - Lipid oxidation and inflammation

Enhanced platelet activity may accentuate a prothrombotic state. Although abnormalities in platelet function have not been well quantified in patients with the metabolic syndrome, an increased susceptibility has been reported for various conditions. Cigarette smokers seem prone to increased platelet aggregation.[69] Several studies indicate that platelet dysfunction is typical of diabetic and obese patients.[70-72] Finally, platelets can be activated by the microinflammation characteristic of the metabolic syndrome.[73] These abnormalities provide a rationale for use of antiplatelet drugs to reduce risk for atherosclerotic cardiovascular disease (ASCVD) in patients with the metabolic syndrome.

Proinflammatory State

Patients with the metabolic syndrome appear to be in a state of accelerated atherogenesis, which is an inflammatory process. Such is reflected by the presence of inflammatory cells in the arterial wall—notably, macrophages, neutrophils, and T-lymphocytes. It is also reflected by the presence of elevations of C-reactive protein (CRP). The liver produces CRP and other acute-phase reactants in response to exposure to excess cytokines. Thus, high levels of CRP reflect a proinflammatory state. Whether the site of chronic inflammation is limited to the arterial wall in patients with the metabolic syndrome is uncertain. This section will focus on atherogenic causes of a proinflammatory state. It will also speculate about the possibility that chronic inflammation exists in other sites as well.

There are three major causes of a state of chronic inflammation: tissue injury, tissue response to injury, and heightened response to injury produced by acute-phase reactants (Table 3-5).

Arterial Injury as a Cause of Arterial Inflammation

All of the risk factors (cigarette smoking, high levels of apo B-containing lipoproteins, low HDL, hypertension, hyperglycemia, and a prothrombotic state) presumably initiate a state of chronic inflammation in the arterial wall. The mechanisms for these effects have been extensively studied and are reviewed in Chapter 2.

Arterial Response to Risk-Factor Injury

In response to risk-factor injury, the arterial wall produces an influx of inflammatory cells. These cells include primarily macrophages but also neutrophils and T-lymphocytes. They act to limit the injury. For example, macrophages ingest modified lipoproteins in an effort to remove injurious lipids. In the process, they are transformed into foam cells. These more acute inflammatory cells release products that elicit smooth muscle proliferation, which in turn causes collagen secretion and converts the atheroma into a fibrous plaque. It is possible that overly robust responses to injury, possibly genetically based, cause accelerated atherosclerosis and contribute to premature ASCVD. When macrophages in the arterial wall are activated, they release cytokines that activate partner inflammatory cells. Some of these cytokines presumably leak into the circulation, where the liver recognizes them as a signal to initiate the formation of acute-phase reactants.

Enhancement of Arterial Inflammation
by Acute-phase Reactants

In response to cytokines derived from the arterial wall, the liver produces several acute-phase reactants, including CRP, fibrinogen, and serum amyloid A. These factors are designed to enhance the arterial wall inflammation, which accelerates the atherogenic process.

Enhancement of Arterial Inflammation by Cytokines

Obese persons and/or those resistant to insulin have high circulating levels of cytokines released from adipose and possibly other tissues (eg, muscle and liver). These cytokines could directly enhance the arterial wall response to injury, or they could act indirectly through enhanced release of acute-phase reactants by the liver.

Metabolic Syndrome as a Generalized Proinflammatory State

This description of steps in the inflammatory process indicates that persons with the metabolic syndrome are in a proinflammatory state. Possibly, this state extends to other organs and might be responsible for other abnormalities, such as insulin resistance and nonalcoholic steatohepatitis.

Summary

The metabolic syndrome is a multifactorial condition requiring interaction of upstream and downstream abnormalities. Without one or the other defect, the syndrome will not develop. Upstream abnormalities can be either obesity or insulin resistance, either primary or acquired. Downstream defects can arise in the regulation of any of the components of the syndrome. Many potential polymorphisms in genes regulating risk factors can contribute to the metabolic syndrome. Only a small portion of these polymorphisms has been elucidated.

In the general population, obesity is the driving force behind the metabolic syndrome. Even when genetic aberrations are present, the metabolic syndrome usually does not develop without the coexistence of obesity. This holds true whether the genetic abnormalities are in insulin signaling or in individual risk factors. Even in populations with a high prevalence of primary insulin resistance, complications rarely develop in persons without excess body fat. The increasing prevalence of the metabolic syndrome in the United States can be explained by the rise in prevalence of obesity.

There has been great interest in insulin resistance as the cause of the metabolic syndrome. Some investigators use the term 'insulin resistance syndrome' for the clustering of metabolic risk factors. This term adds confusion by including obesity as a cause of insulin resistance. Though obesity does cause insulin resistance, it is almost certain that obesity has multiple detrimental effects on pathways of metabolic risk factors that are independent of insulin resistance. Nonetheless, the presence of insulin resistance independent of obesity can also elicit the metabolic syndrome when concomitant metabolic defects are present. Essentially, primary insulin resistance recapitulates the effects of obesity on metabolism. This effect is accentuated with the additional presence of some degree of obesity.

Despite views to the contrary, insulin resistance per se is not synonymous with the metabolic syndrome, which is defined by multiple metabolic risk factors. Their combination explains why lifestyle change (weight reduction and increased physical activity) may not be sufficient to reverse the syndrome.

References

1.   Grundy SM, Mok HY, Zech L, et al: Transport of very low density lipoprotein triglycerides in varying degrees of obesity and hypertriglyceridemia. *J Clin Invest* 1979;63:1274-1283.

2.   Egusa G, Beltz WF, Grundy SM, et al: Influence of obesity on the metabolism of apolipoprotein B in humans. *J Clin Invest* 1985;76:596-603.

3.   Kesaniemi YA, Beltz WF, Grundy SM: Comparisons of metabolism of apolipoprotein B in normal subjects, obese patients, and patients with coronary heart disease. *J Clin Invest* 1985;76:586-595.

4.   McGarry JD, Foster DW: Regulation of hepatic fatty acid oxidation and ketone body production. *Annu Rev Biochem* 1980;49: 395-420.

5.   Vockley J, Singh RH, Whiteman DA: Diagnosis and management of defects of mitochondrial beta-oxidation. *Curr Opin Clin Nutr Metab Care* 2002;5:601-609.

6.   Gehrisch S: Common mutations of the lipoprotein lipase gene and their clinical significance. *Curr Atheroscler Rep* 1999;1:70-78.

7.   Santamarina-Fojo S: The familial chylomicronemia syndrome. *Endocrinol Metab Clin North Am* 1998;27:551-567.

8.   Shachter NS: Apolipoproteins C-I and C-III as important modulators of lipoprotein metabolism. *Curr Opin Lipidol* 2001; 12:297-304.

9.   Alaupovic P, Mack WJ, Knight-Gibson C, et al: The role of triglyceride-rich lipoprotein families in the progression of atherosclerotic lesions as determined by sequential coronary angiography from a controlled clinical trial. *Arterioscler Thromb Vasc Biol* 1997;17:715-722.

10.   Mahley RW, Weisgraber KH, Innerarity TL, et al: Genetic defects in lipoprotein metabolism. Elevation of atherogenic lipoproteins caused by impaired catabolism. *JAMA* 1991;265: 78-83.

11.   Pennacchio LA, Rubin EM: Apolipoprotein a5, a newly identified gene that affects plasma triglyceride levels in humans and mice. *Arterioscler Thromb Vasc Biol* 2003;23:529-534.

12.   Hobbs HH, Brown MS, Goldstein JL: Molecular genetics of the LDL receptor gene in familial hypercholesterolemia. *Hum Mutat* 1992;1:445-466.

13.   Grundy SM, Vega GL: Causes of high blood cholesterol. *Circulation* 1990;81:412-427.

14.   Denke MA, Sempos CT, Grundy SM: Excess body weight. An underrecognized contributor to high blood cholesterol levels in white American men. *Arch Intern Med* 1993;153:1093-1103.

15.   Vega GL, Grundy SM: Hypoalphalipoproteinemia (low high density lipoprotein) as a risk factor for coronary heart disease. *Curr Opin Lipidol* 1996;7:209-216.

16.   Connelly PW, Hegele RA: Hepatic lipase deficiency. *Crit Rev Clin Lab Sci* 1998;35:547-572.

17.   Blades B, Vega GL, Grundy SM: Activities of lipoprotein lipase and hepatic triglyceride lipase in postheparin plasma of patients with low concentrations of HDL cholesterol. *Arterioscler Thromb* 1993;13:1227-1235.

18. Nie L, Wang J, Clark LT, et al: Body mass index and hepatic lipase gene (LIPC) polymorphism jointly influence postheparin plasma hepatic lipase activity. *J Lipid Res* 1998;39:1127-1130.

19. Deeb SS, Zambon A, Carr MC, et al: Hepatic lipase and dyslipidemia: interactions among genetic variants, obesity, gender, and diet. *J Lipid Res* 2003;44:1279-1286.

20. Shohet RV, Vega GL, Bersot TP, et al: Sources of variability in genetic association studies: insights from the analysis of hepatic lipase (LIPC). *Hum Mutat* 2002;19:536-542.

21. Barter PJ, Brewer HB Jr, Chapman MJ, et al: Cholesteryl ester transfer protein: a novel target for raising HDL and inhibiting atherosclerosis. *Arterioscler Thromb Vasc Biol* 2003;23:160-167.

22. Brewer HB Jr, Santamarina-Fojo S: Clinical significance of high-density lipoproteins and the development of atherosclerosis: focus on the role of the adenosine triphosphate-binding cassette protein A1 transporter. *Am J Cardiol* 2003;92:10K-16K.

23. Attie AD, Kastelein JP, Hayden MR: Pivotal role of ABCA1 in reverse cholesterol transport influencing HDL levels and susceptibility to atherosclerosis. *J Lipid Res* 2001;42:1717-1726.

24. *Seventh Report of the Joint National Committee on Prevention, Detection, Evaluation, and Treatment of High Blood Pressure.* US Department of Health and Human Services. National Institutes of Health. National Heart, Lung, and Blood Institute. May 2003. NIH Publication No. 03-5233.

25. Hall JE: The kidney, hypertension, and obesity. *Hypertension* 2003;41:625-633.

26. Hall JE: Mechanisms of abnormal renal sodium handling in obesity hypertension. *Am J Hypertens* 1997;10:49S-55S.

27. Hall JE, Hildebrandt DA, Kuo J: Obesity hypertension: role of leptin and sympathetic nervous system. *Am J Hypertens* 2001; 14:103S-115S.

28. Ferrannini E, Natali A: Essential hypertension, metabolic disorders, and insulin resistance. *Am Heart J* 1991;121:1274-1282.

29. Reaven G: Insulin resistance, hypertension, and coronary heart disease. *J Clin Hypertens (Greenwich)* 2003;5:269-274.

30. Appel LJ: Lifestyle modification as a means to prevent and treat high blood pressure. *J Am Soc Nephrol* 2003;14:S99-S102.

31. Plante GE: Impact of aging on the body's vascular system. *Metabolism* 2003;52:31-35.

32. Lifton RP, Gharavi AG, Geller DS: Molecular mechanisms of human hypertension. *Cell* 2001;104:545-556.

33. Rice T, Rankinen T, Chagnon YC, et al: Genomewide linkage scan of resting blood pressure: HERITAGE Family Study. Health, Risk Factors, Exercise Training, and Genetics. *Hypertension* 2002;39:1037-1043.

34. von Wowern F, Bengtsson K, Lindgren CM, et al: A genome wide scan for early onset primary hypertension in Scandinavians. *Human Mol Genet* 2003;12:2077-2081.

35. Cooper RS, Luke A, Zhu X, et al: Genome scan among Nigerians linking blood pressure to chromosomes 2, 3, and 19. *Hypertension* 2002;40:629-633.

36. Lovati E, Ferrari P, Dick B, et al: Molecular basis of human salt sensitivity: the role of the 11beta-hydroxysteroid dehydrogenase type 2. *J Clin Endocrinol Metab* 1999;84:3745-3749.

37. Bianchi G, Tripodi G: Genetics of hypertension: the adducin paradigm. *Ann N Y Acad Sci* 2003;986:660-668.

38. Siffert W: G-protein beta3 subunit 825T allele and hypertension. *Curr Hypertens Rep* 2003;5:47-53.

39. Jose PA, Eisner GM, Felder RA: Dopamine receptor-coupling defect in hypertension. *Curr Hypertens Rep* 2002;4:237-244.

40. Baudin B: Angiotensin II receptor polymorphisms in hypertension. Pharmacogenomic considerations. *Pharmacogenomics* 2002;3:65-73.

41. Pravenec M, Kurtz TW: Genetics of Cd36 and the hypertension metabolic syndrome. *Semin Nephrol* 2002;22:148-153.

42. Sesti G: Apoptosis in the beta cells: cause or consequence of insulin secretion defect in diabetes? *Ann Med* 2002;34:444-450.

43. Herchuelz A, Diaz-Horta O, van Eylen F: Na/Ca exchange and Ca2+ homeostasis in the pancreatic beta-cell. *Diabetes Metab* 2002;28:3S54-3S60.

44. LeRoith D: Beta-cell dysfunction and insulin resistance in type 2 diabetes: role of metabolic and genetic abnormalities. *Am J Med* 2002;113:3S-11S.

45. Porte D Jr, Kahn SE: Beta-cell dysfunction and failure in type 2 diabetes: potential mechanisms. *Diabetes* 2001;50:S160-S163.

46. Garg A, Chandalia M, Vuitch F: Severe islet amyloidosis in congenital generalized lipodystrophy. *Diabetes Care* 1996;19:28-31.

47. Chang AM, Halter JB: Aging and insulin secretion. *Am J Physiol Endocrinol Metab* 2003;284:E7-E12.

48. Porte D Jr, Kahn SE: Beta-cell dysfunction and failure in type 2 diabetes: potential mechanisms. *Diabetes* 2001;50:S160-S163.

49. Porte D Jr: Clinical importance of insulin secretion and its interaction with insulin resistance in the treatment of type 2 diabetes mellitus and its complications. *Diabetes Metab Res Rev* 2001; 17:181-188.

50. Porte D Jr: Banting lecture 1990. Beta-cells in type II diabetes mellitus. *Diabetes* 1991;40:166-180.

51. Purrello F, Rabuazzo AM: Metabolic factors that affect beta-cell function and survival. *Diabetes Nutr Metab* 2000;13:84-91.

52. De Pergola G, Pannacciulli N: Coagulation and fibrinolysis abnormalities in obesity. *J Endocrinol Invest* 2002;25:899-904.

53. Juhan-Vague I, Alessi MC, Mavri A: Plasminogen activator inhibitor-1, inflammation, obesity, insulin resistance and vascular risk. *J Thromb Haemost* 2003;1:1575-1579.

54. Alessi MC, Morange P, Juhan-Vague I: Fat cell function and fibrinolysis. *Horm Metab Res* 2000;32:504-508.

55. Alessi MC, Bastelica D, Mavri A, et al: Plasma PAI-1 levels are more strongly related to liver steatosis than to adipose tissue accumulation. *Arterioscler Thromb Vasc Biol* 2003;23:1262-1268.

56. Bastard JP, Pieroni L, Hainque B: Relationship between plasma plasminogen activator inhibitor 1 and insulin resistance. *Diabetes Metab Res Rev* 2000;16:192-201.

57. Nakamura T, Adachi H, Hirai Y, et al: Association of plasminogen activator inhibitor-1 with insulin resistance in Japan where obesity is rare. *Metabolism* 2003;52:226-229.

58. Huber K, Christ G, Wojta J, et al: Plasminogen activator inhibitor type-1 in cardiovascular disease. Status report 2001. *Thromb Res* 2001;103:S7-S19.

59. Nordt TK, Lohrmann J, Bode C: Regulation of PAI-1 expression by genetic polymorphisms. Impact on atherogenesis. *Thromb Res* 2001;103:S1-S5.

60. Andersen P: Hypercoagulability and reduced fibrinolysis in hyperlipidemia: relationship to the metabolic cardiovascular syndrome. *J Cardiovasc Pharmacol* 1992;20:S29-S31.

61. Tsiara S, Elisaf M, Mikhailidis DP: Influence of smoking on predictors of vascular disease. *Angiology* 2003;54:507-530.

62. Haffner SM: Insulin resistance, inflammation, and the prediabetic state. *Am J Cardiol* 2003;92:18J-26J.

63. Esmon CT: Does inflammation contribute to thrombotic events? *Haemostasis* 2000;30:34-40.

64. Iacoviello L, Vischetti M, Zito F, et al: Genes encoding fibrinogen and cardiovascular risk. *Hypertension* 2001;38:1199-1203.

65. Miller GJ: Lipoproteins and the haemostatic system in atherothrombotic disorders. *Baillières Clin Haematol* 1994;7:713-732.

66. Glowinska B, Urban M, Koput A, et al: New atherosclerosis risk factors in obese, hypertensive and diabetic children and adolescents. *Atherosclerosis* 2003;167:275-286.

67. Niessner A, Graf S, Nikfardjam M, et al: Circulating t-PA antigen predicts major adverse coronary events in patients with stable coronary artery disease–a 13-year follow-up. *Thromb Haemost* 2003;90:344-350.

68. Juhan-Vague I, Alessi MC, Vague P: Thrombogenic and fibrinolytic factors and cardiovascular risk in non-insulin-dependent diabetes mellitus. *Ann Med* 1996;28:371-380.

69. Lehr HA: Microcirculatory dysfunction induced by cigarette smoking. *Microcirculation* 2000;7:367-384.

70. Carr ME: Diabetes mellitus: a hypercoagulable state. *J Diabetes Complications* 2001;15:44-54.

71. Vinik AI, Erbas T, Park TS, et al: Platelet dysfunction in type 2 diabetes. *Diabetes Care* 2001;24:1476-1485.

72. Konstantinides S, Schafer K, Loskutoff DJ: The prothrombotic effects of leptin: possible implications for the risk of cardiovascular disease in obesity. *Ann N Y Acad Sci* 2001;947:134-141.

73. Tselepis AD, John Chapman M: Inflammation, bioactive lipids and atherosclerosis: potential roles of a lipoprotein-associated phospholipase A2, platelet activating factor-acetylhydrolase. *Atheroscler Suppl* 2002;3:57-68.

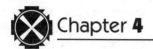

Chapter **4**

Prevalence and Clinical Expression in Populations

Because the metabolic syndrome has so many components and is so variably expressed in populations, the most accurate appreciation of its enormous burden will come from a broad view of the prevalence of its major components, added to educated estimates of the occurrence of the entire syndrome.

Obesity and Overweight

Obesity is defined as a body mass index (BMI) greater than 30 kg/m². Patients with a BMI between 25 and 29.9 are considered overweight. During the past 20 years, the weight of United States citizens has dramatically increased.[1] In 2000, 38.8 million American adults were obese. Twenty states have obesity prevalence rates of 15% to 19%; 29 states have rates of 20% to 24%; and one state, Mississippi, reports a rate of more than 25%. This represents an increase in defined obesity of 61% since 1991. Between 1991 and 1998, seven states reported an increase in obesity of 75%. An equal percentage of the population is overweight but does not qualify as obese. The rate of obesity is still rising: between 2000 and 2001, obesity prevalence climbed from 19.9% to 20.9% (Table 4-1). As of 2003, there were 44 million obese American adults,

74% more than in 1991. Men and women are equally affected. Age is generally proportional to weight, with an exception for the elderly, perhaps because of obesity-related mortality. Blacks are heavier than Hispanics, who are heavier than whites. In 1991, 49% of black women had a BMI of more than 27.3 kg/m^2. A lower level of education is associated with greater body fat, and smokers are less likely to be obese.[1-3]

The problem is not limited to the United States. The World Health Organization (WHO) has identified obesity as a global epidemic (Table 4-2).[4,5]

Europe

Current prevalence data from individual national studies suggest that the prevalence of obesity in European countries ranges from 10% to 20% for men and from 10% to 25% for women. The prevalence of obesity has increased substantially in most European countries in the past 10 years. The most dramatic increase has been in the United Kingdom, where it has more than doubled since 1980. However, there is some evidence that this trend is leveling off among women, at least in some Scandinavian countries.[5]

Africa

In contrast to most Western countries, the emphasis in Africa has been on undernutrition and food scarcity rather than overweight and obesity, so there are few data on current obesity prevalence. However, regional studies indicate a growing prevalence of overweight and obesity in certain socioeconomic groups.

The Middle East

The limited data available indicate that the prevalence of obesity in Middle Eastern countries is high, particularly in women, who appear, in general, to have a higher prevalence of obesity than women in most Western countries.[5] According to a WHO survey, 24% of women and 16% of men in Saudi Arabia were obese, as were 44% of women and 32% of men in Kuwait.[5]

The Caribbean and South America

Obesity is a significant problem in the Caribbean, particularly in countries with a higher per capita gross national product, and it affects women more than men. Brazil is the only Latin American country to have a nationally representative survey conducted in the last 10 years. The PNSN survey indicated that obesity is prevalent in Brazil and is rising, especially among lower-income groups. The problem of dietary deficit appears to be rapidly shifting to one of dietary excess.[6]

Western Pacific

Obesity has long been regarded by Polynesian and Micronesian societies of the Pacific region as a symbol of high social status and prosperity. Its prevalence has risen dramatically in the last 20 years. In 1991, more than 75% of urban males in Western Samoa were classified as obese.

Far East

In Japan, obesity in men has doubled since 1982; in women, its rise has been restricted to a younger age group (20 to 29 years), in whom it has increased 180% since 1976. In the National Nutrition Survey of 1990-1994, less than 3% of the population was classified as obese, with approximately 24.3% of men and 20.2% of women classified as overweight.[7]

The Republic of Korea's National Nutrition Survey of 1995 found that only 1.5% of the population was classified as obese and that 20.5% were overweight. In Thailand, 4% were obese and 16% were overweight. In Malaysia, 4.7% of men and 7.7% of women were obese.[8]

Obesity is increasing in China and is more common in urban areas and among women. In China's National Nutrition Survey of 1992, low rates of obesity were found among men and women (<2%). In urban regions (excluding Beijing, Shanghai, and Tianjin), the prevalence of overweight was 12.3% of men and 14.4% of women (comparable figures for rural regions were 5.3% and 9.8%).[9]

Table 4-1: Prevalence of Obesity in US Adults

Characteristics	Percentage Obese*	
	1991	**1995**
Total (in percentage)	12.0	15.3
Gender		
Men	11.7	15.6
Women	12.2	15.0
Age groups		
18-29	7.1	10.1
30-39	11.3	14.4
40-49	15.8	17.9
50-59	16.1	21.6
60-69	14.7	19.4
>70	11.4	12.1
Race, ethnicity		
White, non-Hispanic	11.3	14.5
Black, non-Hispanic	19.3	22.6
Hispanic	11.6	16.8
Other	7.3	9.6
Educational level		
Less than high school	16.5	20.1
High school degree	13.3	16.7
Some college	10.7	15.1
College or above	8.0	11.0
Smoking status		
Never smoked	12.0	15.2
Ex-smoker	14.0	17.9
Current smoker	9.9	12.3

*Behavioral Risk Factor Surveillance System data by year.
National Center for Chronic Disease Prevention and
Health Promotion. 1991-2001 prevalence of obesity

Percentage Obese*			
1998	**1999**	**2000**	**2001**
17.9	18.9	19.8	20.9
17.7	19.1	20.2	21.0
18.1	18.6	19.4	20.8
12.1	12.1	13.5	14.0
16.9	18.6	20.2	20.5
21.2	22.4	22.9	24.7
23.8	24.2	25.6	26.1
21.3	22.3	22.9	25.3
14.6	16.1	15.5	17.1
16.6	17.7	18.5	19.6
26.9	27.3	29.3	31.1
20.8	21.5	23.4	23.7
11.9	12.4	12.0	15.7
24.1	25.3	26.1	27.4
19.4	20.6	21.7	23.2
17.8	18.1	19.5	21.0
13.1	14.3	15.2	15.7
17.9	19.0	19.9	20.9
20.9	21.5	22.7	23.9
14.8	15.7	16.3	17.8

among US adults, by characteristics. Available from: http://www.cdc.gov/nccdphp/dnpa/obesity/trend/ prev_char.htm. Accessed September 16, 2003.

Table 4-2: Obesity Prevalence Worldwide (BMI >30)

Country/ Region	Year	Age (years)	Men (percentage)	Women (percentage)
Canada	1991	18-74	15	15
Québec	1998	20-64	13.5	11.7
South Africa— Cape Peninsular	1990	15-64	8	44
Ghana	1987/8	20+	0.9	–
Saudi Arabia	1990-93	15+		
Total		16	24	
Urban		18	28	
Rural		12	18	
Kuwait	1994	18+	32	44
West Germany	1991	25-69	16	21
Netherlands	1994	20-59	10	11
Australia	1989	20-69	9.3	11.1
Japan	1993	20+	1.7	2.7
Czech Republic	1988	20-65	16	20

BMI = body mass index

International Association for the Study of Obesity. International Obesity Task Force (Web site). Available from http://www.iotf.org. Accessed September 16, 2003.

Prevalence in Children

More than 25% of US children are overweight. In some European countries, childhood obesity is approaching or has exceeded US levels. Germany and Italy each have a prevalence of approximately 35% in 10-year-old children.

The level in France is about 20%, and in the United Kingdom, it is about 15%.

In China, about 10% of schoolchildren were obese in 1992.[9] Recent data from Japanese schoolchildren 6 to 14 years of age show the prevalence of obesity ranging between 5% and 11%.[10]

Physical Inactivity

Inactivity increases the relative risk of coronary artery disease by a factor between 1.5 and 2.4, equivalent to smoking, hypertension, or elevated blood cholesterol. In 1998, the American Heart Association reported that 29% of US adults participate in no leisure-time physical activity, 44% do inadequate amounts, and only 27% achieve the recommended level. The highest prevalence of recommended activity is among educated, high-income, young white males living in the Western states.[11] Improvement is not on the horizon; high-school participation in physical education classes fell from 42% in 1991 to 29.1% in 1999.[12,13]

Sedentary lifestyles have received far less attention worldwide than their impact on health merits. The WHO attributes 2 million deaths per year to physical inactivity and warns that a sedentary lifestyle might qualify as 1 of the 10 leading causes of death and disability in the world. According to the WHO, 60% to 85% of people in the world, regardless of socioeconomic status, are insufficiently active, including nearly two thirds of children.[14]

Metabolic Syndrome

The prevalence of the metabolic syndrome in many Western countries is 25% to 35%. Hansen[15] estimated the global prevalence of the metabolic syndrome in adults to be about 35%, based on an approximate prevalence of abnormal glucose metabolism, obesity, and insulin resistance.

People with low birth weight (or more specifically, thinness at birth) who become obese as adults are at particularly high risk of the metabolic syndrome in later life, producing a high prevalence in communities with poor fetal nutrition.[16]

United States

Researchers at the Centers for Disease Control and Prevention (CDC) have estimated that as many as 47 million people in the United States (22% to 23% of the population) have the metabolic syndrome.[17] Analysis of data from a 1988-1994 national health survey found prevalence rates ranging from 27.2% of Mexican-American women to 13.9% of black men. Among black women, 20.9% qualified for a diagnosis of metabolic syndrome, as did 22.9% of white women. The rate among Mexican-American men was 20.8%; among white men, it was 24.3%.[18,19] As with obesity, the prevalence increases from 7% for adults 20 to 30 years of age to more than 40% for adults more than 60 years of age.[20]

Europe

The European Group for the Study of Insulin Resistance collected data from euglycemic insulin clamp studies in approximately 1,500 hyperinsulinemic whites from 21 clinical centers all over Europe. Using the definition of metabolic syndrome proposed by the WHO expert committee, they found the prevalence of the metabolic syndrome in healthy whites to be 15.6%, with fewer than 1% of the population having all the components of the syndrome.[21]

Asia-Pacific

In India, the presence of components of the metabolic syndrome is strongly related to socioeconomic status. Between a lower-income segment and a higher-income segment from the same region in southern India, rates were 40% to 280% higher in the more affluent group.[22]

People in Asia, including Hong Kong and parts of mainland China, have experienced a lower incidence of components of the metabolic syndrome than comparable Western populations. However, an alarmingly rapid increase is being found, particularly in younger age groups. Studies in Hong Kong suggest that the risk in a Chinese population starts to increase at a BMI greater than 22 kg/m^2, suggesting that the criteria may be need to be redefined.[23]

Cardiovascular death rates and the prevalence of hypertension have been compared between populations of Chinese, Malays, and Indians in Singapore and populations in Wales, England, Japan, and the United States. Mortality from ischemic heart disease was found to be highest in the Indian population, followed by the Malay, Western, Chinese, and Japanese groups. Mortality from cerebrovascular disease was highest in the Malay population, followed in order by the Indian, Chinese, Japanese, English, Welsh, and US populations. For hypertension, the order was Malay, Indian, Chinese, US, English, Welsh, and Japanese groups.[24]

Impaired Glucose Tolerance

In 2002, the WHO published an exhaustive listing of impaired glucose tolerance (IGT) prevalence by country and ethnic origin.[25] The prevalence of IGT varied widely among different ethnic groups and incomes and between the sexes.

Although the prevalence of IGT in children of normal weight has yet to be determined,[26] obese children have a high incidence of IGT. Of 167 obese children in a recent study,[27] 55 (25%) of the 4- to 10-year-old age group and 112 (21%) of the adolescents (11 to 18 years of age) had IGT. Silent type 2 diabetes was present in 4% of the obese adolescents. Subjects with IGT had markedly elevated insulin and C-peptide levels after the glucose-tolerance test, but in adolescents with diabetes, the 30-minute insulin: glucose ratio of change was reduced. After controlling for BMI, the best predictor of IGT was insulin resistance, which was greater in the affected cohort.

Diabetes

Of the world's estimated 120 million patients with type 2 diabetes, 30 million are in the Asia-Pacific region. Five of the 10 countries with the highest populations of diabetic patients are in Asia. By 2010, it is predicted that a total of 216 million people worldwide will have type 2 diabetes and that 130 million of these will live in the Asia-Pacific region.[28] India and China are, and will remain through 2025, the countries with the most cases of diabetes mellitus. India is projected to have a diabetic population of 57 million in 2025. China, despite its much greater overall population, will have roughly 38 million diabetic people.[29]

United States

Studies in the heterogeneous US population are capable of wide variations in results but allow for distinctions other than racial and ethnic ones, such as the clear difference between men and women and the increasing incidence of the metabolic syndrome with age. Table 4-3[30] presents the 2003 National Institute of Diabetes and Digestive and Kidney Diseases data on the incidence of diabetes in the United States by group. Because 90% of patients with diabetes have type 2 diabetes, the figures closely parallel the relative incidence of the metabolic syndrome. These data and those from the Pathobiological Determinants of Atherosclerosis in Youth study[31] clearly demonstrate the stronger influence of adiposity on coronary atherosclerosis in men. It is also apparent that men are more prone to abdominal ('android') obesity than women, probably due to higher levels of androgenic hormones. Other studies identify blacks of African origin as prone to hypertension when they gain weight and to type 2 diabetes, possibly because of a relatively low reserve for insulin secretion. On the other hand, blacks of African origin develop less atherogenic dyslipidemia than do whites with the same degree of weight gain.

Hispanics and Native Americans

Hispanics and Native Americans are especially susceptible to type 2 diabetes, but they are less likely to develop hypertension than are blacks. An isolated population in the Southwestern United States, the Pima Indian tribe near Phoenix, Arizona, has an extraordinarily high genetic pre-

Table 4-3: Prevalence of Diabetes in the United States

Population group	Total	Percentage of group
Age ≥20 years	16.9 million	8.6
Age ≥65 years	7 million	20.1
Men	7.8 million	8.3
Women	9.1 million	8.9
Age <20 years	151,000	0.19
Non-Hispanic whites	11.4 million	7.8
Non-Hispanic blacks	2.8 million	13
Hispanic/ Latino Americans	2 million	10.2
Native Americans and Alaska Natives*	105,000	15.1
Alaska Natives		(5.3)
Native Americans in southeastern United States		(25.7)
Pima Indians (30-60 years of age)	7,000	50
Native Hawaiians		15.5
Total	17 million	

* who receive care from the Indian Health Service (IHS)

National Institute of Diabetes and Digestive and Kidney Diseases: National diabetes statistics. NIH Publication no. 03-3892. May 2003. Available from: http:// diabetes.niddk.nih.gov/health/diabetes/pubs/dmstats/ dmstats.htm#9. Accessed September 17, 2003.

disposition to cholelithiasis, type 2 diabetes, insulin resistance, and obesity.[32]

Europe

The Mediterranean Group for the Study of Diabetes[33] estimates that an epidemic expansion will occur in all European countries. It notes that the reported prevalence of diabetes in adults in Italy at least 20 years of age was 7.5% in 1995 and 7.8% in 2000, and it predicts that the prevalence will be 10% in 2025. In Spain, the prevalence of diabetes is projected to rise from 7.2% in 1995 to 9.5% in 2025. More moderate increases are expected in France and Croatia over this period: from 2.1% to 2.6% in France and from 4.4% to 5.1% in Croatia.

South Asia

As a population, Southeast Asians, studied mostly in India, have little tolerance for excess body fat.[34] Risk begins to rise at a BMI of about 23 kg/m.[2,35-37] Undoubtedly, there is individual variability, but South Asians commonly develop insulin resistance with only moderate weight gain.[38] This predisposition commonly appears when South Asians become relatively affluent or migrate to other regions and take up a new lifestyle.[39] The increased risk for coronary heart disease (CHD) in South Asians is roughly double the level that can be explained by standard risk factors.[40] This observation supports the concept that emerging risk factors, which are secondary to overweight, also contribute to CHD risk.

References

1. National Center for Chronic Disease Prevention and Health Promotion: U.S. obesity trends 1985 to 2001. Available from: http://www.cdc.gov/nccdphp/dnpa/obesity/trend/maps/index.htm. Accessed September 16, 2003.

2. Mokdad AH, Bowman BA, Ford ES, et al: The continuing epidemics of obesity and diabetes in the United States. *JAMA* 2001; 286:1195-1200.

3. Mokdad AH, Serdula MK, Dietz WH, et al: The spread of the obesity epidemic in the United States, 1991-1998. *JAMA* 1999;282: 1519-1522.

4.   World Health Organization: *Obesity: Preventing and Managing the Global Epidemic.* Geneva, WHO, 1998.

5.   International Association for the Study of Obesity: International Obesity Task Force Web site. Available from: http://www.iotf.org/. Accessed September 16, 2003.

6.   Mondini L, Monteiro CA: The stage of nutrition transition in different Brazilian regions. *Arch Latinoam Nutr* 1997;47(2 suppl 1): 17-21.

7.   Yoshiike N, Matsumura Y, Zaman MM, et al: Descriptive epidemiology of body mass index in Japanese adults in a representative sample from the National Nutrition Survey 1990-1994. *Int J Obes Relat Metab Disord* 1998;22:684-687.

8.   Ismail MN, Chee SS, Nawawi H, et al: Obesity in Malaysia. *Obes Rev* 2002;3:203-208.

9.   Chen CM: Nutrition status of the Chinese people. *Biomed Environ Sci* 1996;9:81-92.

10.   Kotani K, Nishida M, Yamashita S, et al: Two decades of annual medical examinations in Japanese obese children: do obese children grow into obese adults? *Int J Obes Relat Metab Disord* 1997;21:912-921.

11.   American Heart Association: Physical inactivity. Biostatistical Fact Sheet—Risk Factors. Available from: http://www.americanheart.org/. Accessed September 16, 2003.

12.   Kann L, Kinchen SA, Williams BI, et al: Youth risk behavior surveillance—United States, 1997. *MMWR CDC Surveill Summ* 1998;47:1-89.

13.   Kann L, Kinchen SA, Williams BI, et al: Youth risk behavior surveillance—United States, 1999. *MMWR CDC Surveill Summ* 2000;47:1-32.

14.   World Health Organization: Physical inactivity a leading cause of disease and disability, warns WHO [press release]. Available from: http://www.who.int/inf/en/pr-2002-23.html. Accessed September 16, 2003.

15.   Hansen BC: Genetics of insulin action. *Baillieres Clin Endocrinol Metab* 1993;7:1033-1061.

16.   Hales CN, Barker DJ: Type 2 (non-insulin-dependent) diabetes mellitus: the thrifty phenotype hypothesis. *Diabetologia* 1992;35:595-601.

17.   National Center for Chronic Disease Prevention and Health Promotion: Prevalence among U.S. adults of a metabolic syndrome

associated with obesity. Findings from the third NHANES survey. Available from: http://www.cdc.gov/nccdphp/dnpa/obesity/trend/metabolic.htm. Accessed September 16, 2003.

18. Study finds ethnic differences among Americans. March 22, 2003. Available from: http://www.obgyn.net/newsheadlines/womens_health-Metabolic_Syndrome-20030322-44.asp. Accessed September 16, 2003.

19. Ford ES, Giles WH, Dietz WH: Prevalence of the metabolic syndrome among US adults: findings from the third National Health and Nutrition Examination Survey. *JAMA* 2002;287:356-359.

20. Ford ES, Giles WH: A comparison of the prevalence of the metabolic syndrome using two proposed definitions. *Diabetes Care* 2003;26:575-581.

21. Beck-Nielsen H: General characteristics of the insulin resistance syndrome: prevalence and heritability. The European Group for the Study of Insulin Resistance (EGIR). *Drugs* 1999;58(suppl):7-10.

22. Mohan V, Shanthirani S, Deepa R, et al: Intra-urban differences in the prevalence of the metabolic syndrome in southern India—the Chennai Urban Population Study (CUPS No. 4). *Diabet Med* 2001;18:280-287.

23. Lee ZS, Critchley JA, Chan JC, et al: Obesity in the key determinant of cardiovascular risk factors in the Hong Kong Chinese population: cross-sectional clinic-based study. *Hong Kong Med J* 2000;6:13-23.

24. Hughes K: Mortality from cardiovascular diseases in Chinese, Malays and Indians in Singapore, in comparison with England and Wales, USA and Japan. *Ann Acad Med Singapore* 1989;18:642-645.

25. World Health Organization: Prevalence of impaired glucose tolerance (per cent population) in the age range 30-64 years in the following studied populations. 2002. Available from: http://www.who.int/ncd/dia/databases3.htm. Accessed September 16, 2003.

26. Decsi T, Molnar D: Insulin resistance syndrome in children: pathophysiology and potential management strategies. *Paediatr Drugs* 2003;5:291-299.

27. Sinha R, Fisch G, Teague B, et al: Prevalence of impaired glucose tolerance among children and adolescents with marked obesity. *N Engl J Med* 2002;346:802-810.

28.   Amos AF, McCarty DJ, Zimmet P: The rising global burden of diabetes and its complications: estimates and projections to the year 2010. *Diabet Med* 1997;14(suppl 5):S1-S85.

29.   Roglic G, King H: Diabetes mellitus in Asia [editorial]. *Hong Kong Med J* 2000;6:10-11.

30.   National Institute of Diabetes and Digestive and Kidney Diseases: National diabetes statistics. NIH Publication no. 03-3892. May 2003. Available from: http://diabetes.niddk.nih.gov/health/diabetes/pubs/dmstats/dmstats.htm#9. Accessed September 17, 2003.

31.   McGill HC Jr, McMahan CA, Herderick EE, et al: Obesity accelerates the progression of coronary atherosclerosis in young men. *Circulation* 2002;105:2712-2718.

32.   Howard BV, Lisse JR, Knowler WC, et al: Diabetes and atherosclerosis in the Pima Indians. *Mt Sinai J Med* 1982;49:169-175.

33.   Dalla Vestra M, Crepaldi G: Epidemiology of diabetes mellitus in the north Mediterranean countries. Mediterranean Group for the Study of Diabetes. Available from: http://www.mgsd.net/uk/page5450.asp. Accessed September 16, 2003.

34.   Chambers JC, Eda S, Bassett P, et al: C-reactive protein, insulin resistance, central obesity, and coronary heart disease risk in Indian Asians from the United Kingdom compared with European whites. *Circulation* 2001;104:145-150.

35.   McKeigue PM, Ferrie JE, Pierpoint T, et al: Association of early-onset coronary heart disease in South Asian men with glucose intolerance and hyperinsulinemia. *Circulation* 1993;87:152-161.

36.   Dhawan J: Coronary heart disease risks in Asian Indians. *Curr Opin Lipidol* 1996;7:196-198.

37.   Venkatramana P, Reddy PC: Association of overall and abdominal obesity with coronary heart disease risk factors: comparison between urban and rural Indian men. *Asia Pac J Clin Nutr* 2002;11:66 -71.

38.   Chandalia M, Abate N, Garg A, et al: Relationship between generalized and upper body obesity to insulin resistance in Asian Indian men. *J Clin Endocrinol Metab* 1999;84:2329-2335.

39.   Bhatnagar D, Anand IS, Durrington PN, et al: Coronary risk factors in people from the Indian subcontinent living in west London and their siblings in India. *Lancet* 1995;345:405-409.

40.   Miller GJ, Beckles GL, Maude GH, et al: Ethnicity and other characteristics predictive of coronary heart disease in a developing community: principal results of the St James Survey, Trinidad. *Int J Epidemiol* 1989;18:808-817.

Chapter 5

Associated Clinical Outcomes: Atherosclerotic Cardiovascular Disease and Type 2 Diabetes

Most investigators consider the metabolic syndrome to be a cluster of risk factors for atherosclerotic cardiovascular disease (ASCVD), particularly coronary heart disease (CHD).

Another acknowledged outcome of the metabolic syndrome is type 2 diabetes, which by itself is also a risk factor for ASCVD. Diabetes accelerates atherosclerosis but also causes the small-vessel complications of retinopathy, nephropathy, and neuropathy. Microvascular disease, in addition, may accelerate atherosclerosis. Other associated disorders include nonalcoholic fatty liver disease, polycystic ovary disease, and cholesterol gallstones.

In this chapter, primary emphasis will be on the etiologic role of the metabolic syndrome in ASCVD and type 2 diabetes.

Metabolic Syndrome and ASCVD Risk

If the major outcome of the metabolic syndrome is ASCVD, a key issue is how much risk the syndrome carries for ASCVD. This issue is unresolved. However, a large body of evidence indicates that each component of the metabolic syndrome is accompanied by increased risk for ASCVD. This chapter examines these relationships, both between underlying risk factors and between metabolic risk factors.

Underlying Risk Factors and ASCVD Risk
Overweight/Obesity

Overweight (body mass index [BMI] 25 to 30 kg/m²) and obese (BMI >30 kg/m²) people are at increased risk for ASCVD. The Framingham Heart Study concluded that overweight men were 21% more likely to have cardiovascular disease, and overweight women, 20%. Obese men and women increased their risk to 46% and 64%, respectively, over those of normal weight. Excess weight increased risk for hypertension by 26% in men and 28% in women. It increased risk for angina pectoris by 26% in men and 22% in women, and risk for CHD by 23% in men and 15% in women.[1]

In Harvard's Nurses' Health Study, Wilson et al found similar risk rates among 44,702 women 40 to 65 years of age during 8 years of follow-up. This study found that waist-hip ratio (WHR) and waist circumference independently and significantly increased age-adjusted risk of CHD. A WHR ≥0.76 or waist circumference ≥76.2 cm (30 in) was associated with more than a 2-fold higher risk of CHD, even among women with a BMI of 25 kg/m² or less. A waist circumference ≥96.5 cm (38 in) was associated with a risk ratio of 3.06.[2]

A study from Spain identified preventable causes of death among representative population samples during the 1990s. The study found that 8.5% of all deaths in adults were attributable to excess weight. Almost 70% were cardiovascular deaths, 16% were attributable to tobacco use in adults, and 4% were attributable to hypertension.[3] Dozens of clinical trials have demonstrated positive benefits on cardiovascular risk factors from weight reduction even as modest as 5%.[4-10]

The mechanisms whereby overweight/obesity promotes the risk for ASCVD have not been fully explained. According to the Framingham Heart Study,[11] much of the relationship can be explained by the effects of obesity on the major risk factors—total cholesterol, high-density lipoprotein (HDL), and blood pressure. However, obesity has adverse effects on many of the emerging risk factors as well, eg, triglycerides, insulin resistance, and proinflammatory and prothrombotic processes. Many investigators believe that some of the adverse effect of overweight/obesity on ASCVD risk is mediated through these risk factors.

Physical Inactivity

Physical inactivity is another underlying risk factor for ASCVD. The American Heart Association,[12] the National Cholesterol Education Program (NCEP),[13] and the US Surgeon General[14] list physical inactivity as a major risk factor. Even though assessment of physical activity presents difficulties in data collection and verification, the accumulated body of evidence is convincing.[15] Some of the primary lines of evidence supporting this position are outlined in Table 5-1.

Physical activity may decrease ASCVD risk in multiple ways. Notably, increased physical activity can reduce blood pressure levels[16] and raise HDL levels.[17] It also reduces insulin resistance[18-20] and likely reduces the risk for diabetes.[21] In addition, physical activity improves cardiovascular fitness, which promotes survival associated with major cardiovascular events.[22-25]

Atherogenic Diet

An atherogenic diet accelerates the development of atherosclerosis and predisposes a person to major coronary events. High intake of saturated fats, trans fats, and cholesterol, and deficient intake of fruits and vegetables characterize such a diet. The evidence underlying a causative relationship between dietary fats and lipids and ASCVD has been extensively reviewed in guideline reports—the NCEP

Table 5-1: Evidence Supporting Physical Inactivity as a Risk Factor for ASCVD

- The Framingham Heart Study has determined that physical activity results in a 40% reduction in overall mortality and that coronary heart disease (CHD) in sedentary men was three times more prevalent than in active men.[22,26]

- In a 10-year Norwegian study, the risk of stroke in middle-aged and elderly women was nearly double for the least active of what it was for the most active.[23]

- It may be more dangerous to cycle through repeated weight loss/weight gain episodes than to remain obese. A 7-year Texas study of 10,529 men 35 to 57 years of age in the upper 10% to 15% of risk for CHD found a significant relationship between weight variability and all-cause and cardiovascular mortality in all but the heaviest men. The relative risk for all-cause mortality between the first and fourth quartiles was 1.64.[27]

Adult Treatment Panel III (ATP III),[13] American Heart Association dietary guidelines,[28] and Dietary Guidelines for Americans 2000.[29] During the past several decades, Americans have modified fat consumption to reduce serum cholesterol levels and risk for ASCVD. While change represents a major public health accomplishment, dietary consumption of atherogenic fats and cholesterol remains higher than recommended levels. In addition, consumption of fruits and vegetables remains lower than recommended.

An important question is whether diet composition contributes to the epidemic of obesity that is occurring in the United States and worldwide. For many years, the prevailing theory was that high-fat diets promote obesity. The fat calories hidden in calorically dense foods were held to blame. This theory led to recommendations to reduce total dietary fat intake and to replace it with carbohydrate. However, it has now become apparent that carbohydrate replacement is not the solution to the obesity problem. Low-fat, high-carbohydrate diets appear to have the same potential for producing weight gain as do high-fat diets. Moreover, high-carbohydrate diets have metabolic drawbacks. They cause exaggerated postprandial glucose and insulin responses, they raise triglyceride levels, and they reduce HDL-cholesterol levels, as compared to higher-fat diets. For these reasons, many investigators are increasingly skeptical that a low-fat, high-carbohydrate diet is appropriate for patients with the metabolic syndrome.

A more balanced fat intake (ie, 30% to 35% of total calories) appears to be a reasonable compromise for those with the metabolic syndrome. The fat should come mostly from vegetable oils that are low in saturated and trans fatty acids and higher in unsaturated fats. Intake of monounsaturated fatty acids should be about twice that of polyunsaturated fatty acids.[13]

Atherogenic Dyslipidemia and Its Components

Four lipid abnormalities characterize atherogenic dyslipidemia: elevated triglyceride levels (and triglyceride-rich lipoproteins), small low-density lipoprotein (LDL) particles, reduced HDL cholesterol levels, and elevated apolipoprotein B (apo B) levels. Typically, there are multiple lipoprotein defects. Often lipoproteins are not categorically abnormal, although some may be marginally abnormal. Detection of some lipoprotein abnormalities may require methodologies that are not used in routine clinical practice.

Atherogenic dyslipidemia commonly occurs in persons with premature CHD. Most patients with atherogenic dyslipidemia show concurrent abdominal obesity and physical inactivity.[30,31] Most also are insulin resistant.

Atherogenic dyslipidemia is the same as the 'diabetic dys-lipidemia' found in people with type 2 diabetes.[32,33] Al-though attempts have been made in epidemiologic stud-ies to identify the contributions of each component of atherogenic dyslipidemia to CHD risk, the close associa-tion among the factors makes assignment of contribution difficult. Nonetheless, there is considerable evidence from epidemiology, genetic forms of dyslipidemia, and animal studies that each component is independently atherogenic.

Elevated serum triglyceride levels

Several epidemiologic studies report a causal relation-ship between high serum triglyceride levels and CHD inci-dence.[34] Triglyceride levels can be confounded because of correlation with total, LDL, and HDL-cholesterol levels as well as with nonlipid risk factors—obesity, hypertension, diabetes, cigarette smoking, insulin resistance, and prothrombotic state. Thus, a high triglyceride level may signify increased risk for CHD, regardless of whether it is an independent risk factor. In fact, recent meta-analyses of prospective studies strongly suggest that elevated triglyc-eride levels are an independent risk factor for CHD. This finding raises the possibility that some triglyceride-rich li-poproteins (TGRLP) are atherogenic. The issue of inde-pendence of risk should focus more on particular TGRLP than on triglycerides per se.

Lipoprotein remnants as atherogenic lipoproteins

Remnant lipoproteins are cholesterol-enriched particles that have many of the properties of LDL; they consist mostly of small, very low-density lipoprotein (VLDL) and inter-mediate-density lipoprotein (IDL). Growing evidence sup-ports the atherogenicity of these remnants.[35] In experimen-tal animals, they definitely cause atherosclerosis.[36] In humans, some genetic hyperlipidemias manifest remnant accumulation. These disorders commonly produce prema-ture CHD and peripheral vascular disease. In several clini-cal studies, elevated remnants strongly predicted coronary atherosclerosis or CHD.[37-41] Drug therapies that reduce remnant lipoproteins (fibrates, nicotinic acid, and statins) also reduce risk for CHD.[42-45] Overall evidence indicates that remnant lipoproteins are as atherogenic as LDL.

VLDL cholesterol as a marker
for remnant lipoproteins

Remnant lipoproteins include a spectrum of TGRLP. No single test specifically identifies these lipoproteins. VLDL cholesterol nonetheless provides an adequate marker for clinical practice.[13] Most VLDL cholesterol apparently occurs in atherogenic remnants.[46] When serum triglyceride levels are <400 mg/dL, VLDL cholesterol can be estimated as triglyceride divided by 5.

Common causes of elevated triglyceride and VLDL cholesterol levels include overweight and obesity, physical inactivity, cigarette smoking, excess alcohol intake, very high-carbohydrate diets (>60% of total energy), other diseases (type 2 diabetes, chronic renal failure, nephrotic syndrome), and certain drugs (corticosteroids, protease inhibitors for human immunodeficiency virus [HIV], β-adrenergic blocking agents, estrogens).[47,48] These factors often raise triglyceride levels to 150 to 199 mg/dL,[49] and can contribute to even higher levels. But when triglyceride levels are ≥200 mg/dL, genetic abnormalities in triglyceride metabolism usually contribute as well.

The atherogenicity of TGRLP may depend to some extent on the underlying cause. For example, elevations of TGRLP may be more atherogenic when produced by obesity or diabetes and less atherogenic when associated with excess alcohol consumption or estrogen replacement. If differences in atherogenicity exist, they probably relate to the type of TGRLP present (ie, large, triglyceride-rich VLDL or smaller, cholesterol-enriched VLDL).

Categories of serum triglycerides

ATP III adopted the categories of serum triglyceride levels shown in Table 5-2. Borderline triglyceride levels (150 to 199 mg/dL) represent a range in which other metabolic risk factors are commonly present. Triglyceride levels in the range of 200 to 499 mg/dL typically signify the presence of increased remnant lipoproteins. When triglyceride levels exceed 500 mg/dL, the patient is in danger of developing acute pancreatitis. However, acute pancreatitis rarely occurs until triglyceride levels exceed 2,000 mg/dL.

Small LDL Particles

Small LDL particles are another component of atherogenic dyslipidemia. They are associated with increased risk for CHD.[50] However, their specific role in atherogenesis remains to be identified. Detection of small LDL requires special methodology—electrophoresis, nuclear magnetic resonance, or ultracentrifugation. If found, small LDL particles usually indicate multiple abnormalities in lipoprotein metabolism, including elevated triglyceride levels and low HDL levels. LDL cholesterol remains the primary target of treatment in persons with small LDL particles.

Low HDL Cholesterol

ATP III defines as *categorically low* an HDL cholesterol level <40 mg/dL. Low levels of serum HDL cholesterol typically denote increased CHD morbidity and mortality.[11,51] High HDL-cholesterol levels (>60 mg/dL), conversely, suggest reduced risk. Quantitatively, a 1% decrease in HDL cholesterol carries a 2% to 3% increase in CHD risk.[51]

Multiple mechanisms appear to account for the relationship between low HDL and CHD risk. HDL itself carries several potential antiatherogenic properties. It promotes efflux of cholesterol from foam cells in atherosclerotic lesions (reverse cholesterol transport);[52] it retards aggregation of LDL particles; and it possesses antioxidant and anti-inflammatory properties.[53] Moreover, low HDL levels commonly associate with other atherogenic factors. Low levels strongly correlate with elevated serum triglycerides, remnant lipoproteins,[54] and small LDL particles.[55] They further associate strongly with insulin resistance and its associated metabolic risk factors.[55] Therefore, much of the power of low HDL to predict CHD may be independent of its antiatherogenic properties.

Table 5-2: Categories of Serum Triglyceride Levels

Category	Serum Triglyceride Levels (mg/dL)
Normal	Less than 150
Borderline high	150 to 199
High	200 to 499
Very high	≥500

Causes of low HDL cholesterol

Factors contributing to low HDL-cholesterol levels are elevated serum triglyceride levels, overweight and obesity, physical inactivity, cigarette smoking, very high-carbohydrate diets, type 2 diabetes, certain drugs (β-blockers, anabolic steroids, progestational agents), and genetic factors. About half of the variability in HDL-cholesterol levels in the general population comes from genetic factors;[56] the other half arises from acquired factors. Among the latter, overweight and obesity are most important.[57]

Apolipoprotein AI (apo A1) is the major apolipoprotein of HDL. A low apo AI level is associated with increased risk for CHD, although not independently of low HDL. Some investigators suggest that measurement of apo AI provides predictive information. ATP III does not recommend its routine measurement.

Elevated Apolipoprotein B and Non-HDL Cholesterol

All atherogenic lipoproteins carry apolipoprotein B (apo B). Therefore its measurement could be useful for predictive purposes. Its superiority over LDL cholesterol in risk prediction, however, remains unproven.[58] Its greatest utility for prediction lies in patients with elevated triglyceride levels. In such patients, atherogenic lipoproteins often are elevated out of proportion to LDL-cholesterol. Non-HDL cholesterol (VLDL + LDL cholesterol) correlates strongly with total apo B. It is estimated by calculating total cholesterol minus HDL cholesterol, values readily available in clinical practice.[46] In ATP III, non-HDL cholesterol is designated as a secondary target of cholesterol-lowering therapy in persons whose triglyceride levels are ≥200 mg/dL.

Elevated Blood Pressure and ASCVD Risk

Many studies document a powerful association between high blood pressure levels and risk for CHD.[59-62] Elevated blood pressure also increases risk for stroke. Even at less than categoric hypertension (≥140/90 mm Hg), patients with high-normal blood pressure (130 to 139 mm Hg systolic and/or 85 to 89 mm Hg diastolic) carry a higher risk for CHD compared with those with optimal values.[63] For patients with diabetes, the risks appear even greater. Recent estimates suggest that a significant portion of ASCVD in diabetics is due to hypertension and that the risks begin at pressures previously considered 'normal.' Clinical trials have established that lowering blood pressure in hypertensive patients reduces the likelihood for suffering several major cardiovascular disease (CVD) events, including CHD.[64] Older people with isolated systolic hypertension also benefit. Several large population studies have confirmed the benefits of reducing systolic blood pressure levels to less than 130 mm Hg in diabetic patients.[65]

Insulin Resistance and ASCVD Risk

An important question is whether insulin resistance is a risk factor for CHD or other CVD events. Two issues must be distinguished: (1) whether insulin resistance is associated with increased risk for ASCVD, and (2) whether insulin resistance is an independent causative risk factor. Several studies support an association between insulin resistance and ASCVD.

The Helsinki Policemen Study (970 healthy men aged 34 to 64 years), during its 22-year follow-up, found insulin resistance to be the best predictor of coronary artery disease (CAD) (28% increased risk) and stroke (64% increase).[66] Insulin resistance does not, however, appear to be predictive in women.[67]

From another perspective, insulin resistance was present in 82.5% of 40 newly diagnosed Spanish CAD patients.[68] Insulin resistance was determined by two tests— a standard 75-g oral glucose-tolerance test (OGTT) and an insulin suppression test (IST). In the IST, insulin resistance was estimated by determining the steady-state plasma glucose concentrations during the last 60 minutes of a 150-minute constant infusion of glucose, insulin, and somatostatin. Twenty-seven patients had an abnormal OGTT result. Of these, 88.8% had an abnormal IST result, while 69% of the 13 patients with a normal OGTT result had an abnormal IST result. Insulin resistance has been associated with hyperinsulinemia and ASCVD in several studies.[69,70]

Investigators differ on whether insulin resistance is an independent causative risk factor for ASCVD. Some investigators have postulated that hyperinsulinemia promotes development of atherosclerosis. Reaven and others cite evidence that hyperinsulinemia promotes renal salt retention,[71,72] increased plasma triglyceride levels, decreased HDL-cholesterol, hyperuricemia, smaller and denser LDL particles, and higher circulating levels of PAI-1[73]—all promoters of CVD. Ruotolo notes that hyperinsulinemia promotes excess formation of VLDL particles.[74] Imazu and Corry add sympathetic nervous system activation and vascular smooth-muscle cell proliferation to the list of results of elevated plasma insulin and glucose levels.[16,75] Others suggest that insulin resistance in arterial wall cells accelerates atherogenesis by decreasing endothelial cell production of nitric oxide, which inhibits thrombosis, binding of inflammatory cells to the vascular wall, and vascular smooth-muscle cell migration and proliferation. Still other investigators postulate that increased nonesterified fatty acid (NEFA) levels or an excess of other adipokines caused by insulin resistance leads to enhanced atherosclerosis.[76-79]

A further argument maintains that if insulin resistance is directly responsible for the development of other metabolic risk factors (eg, atherogenic dyslipidemia or hypertension), then insulin resistance is an independent causative risk factor. However, because the mechanisms responsible for all of these other metabolic risk factors have not been elucidated, it is difficult to attribute their presence to an independent action of insulin resistance. Reaven et al[71,73] have been major proponents of the central role of insulin resistance in the cause of other metabolic risk factors. For example, Reaven[80] has speculated that hyperinsulinemia, which is secondary to insulin resistance, promotes increased formation of VLDL triglycerides in the liver, which can account for atherogenic dyslipidemia. If these mechanisms can be confirmed through further investigation, a strong case could be made for insulin resistance being an independent causative risk factor for ASCVD.

Hyperglycemia and ASCVD risk

A significant portion of patients with insulin resistance will eventually develop hyperglycemia (type 2 diabetes). A large body of data from prospective and epidemiologic studies indicates that hyperglycemia per se is an independent risk factor for ASCVD.[69,81-85]

Hyperglycemia promotes formation of advanced glycation end products; accumulation of these products in the arterial wall appears to promote atherogenesis.[86] Elevated plasma glucose has been reported to impair endothelial function, which is postulated to accelerate atherosclerosis.[87] It also induces platelet dysfunction, another potential atherogenic change.[88] And by modifying function of macrophages in the arterial wall, hyperglycemia may stimulate inflammatory responses that predispose to major cardiovascular events.[89]

Proinflammatory State and ASVCD Risk

The metabolic syndrome is characterized by elevated levels of C-reactive protein (CRP). A proinflammatory state exists when cells of the immune system (eg, macrophages, neutrophils, T-lymphocytes) are in a state of activation. When activated cells reside within arterial plaques, the likelihood for major cardiovascular events is increased. Some investigators speculate that high levels of CRP in patients with the metabolic syndrome indicate increased arterial inflammation, a precursor of major cardiovascular events. However, this mechanism has not been proved with certainty. The mechanisms underlying elevated CRP in patients with the metabolic syndrome have not been explained. At least three possibilities exist. First, excess adipose tissue is known to produce inflammatory cytokines (ie, IL-1 β, IL-6, interferon-γ, and tumor necrosis factor-α), along with a host of other metabolically active proteins (IL-8, adiponectin, leptin, plasminogen activator inhibitor-1 [PAI-1], prostaglandin E2, prostacyclin, angiopoietin-2, peroxisome proliferator activated receptor-γ, acetylation stimulating protein, cholesterol ester transfer protein [CETP], uncoupling protein-2, macrophage migration inhibitory factor, vascular endothelial growth factor in rats, transforming growth factor-β in mice, and estrogens).[90-93] Adipose tissue-derived cytokines could both increase production of CRP in the liver and activate cells of the immune system in the arterial wall. Second, high levels of NEFA entering both muscle and liver may stimulate production of cytokines,[94] that, in turn, could raise CRP levels. And third, the risk factors of the metabolic syndrome could induce arterial inflammation, which in turn could release cytokines, raising CRP levels.

What is not known is how elevated CRP concentrations relate to increased risk for major cardiovascular events in patients with the metabolic syndrome. Investigations by Ridker et al[95] and others[96,97] indicate that even high-normal levels of CRP carry predictive power for major cardiovascular events. One possibility is that elevated CRP concentrations are only a marker for increased major cardiovascular events. If so, they could reflect release of cytokines by arterial inflammation or by adipose tissue. Release by arterial inflammation would directly indicate the presence of plaques that are subject to rupture or erosion. Release of CRP by adipose tissue would merely indicate the presence of several other metabolic risk factors. It has further been postulated that an elevation of CRP itself could promote arterial inflammation.[98]

Prothrombotic State and ASCVD Risk

The coagulation system is regulated by two opposing actions: (1) activities that promote thrombus formation, and (2) activities that promote fibrinolysis. The former include components of the coagulation cascade. Particularly important are tissue factor, Factor VI, and prothrombin. An imbalance between the two actions creates the prothrombotic state; both an increase in coagulation factors and an inhibition of fibrinolysis cause that imbalance.

Fibrinolysis is promoted by tissue plasminogen activator (t-PA) but is inhibited by PAI-1. When activities of thrombus formation or antifibrinolysis exceed those of fibrinolysis, a patient is said to be in a *prothrombotic state*. Factors that have been implicated in the prothrombotic state are high levels of Factor VII, fibrinogen, and PAI-1.[99] Of these factors, PAI-1 is the most consistently correlated with all components of the insulin resistance syndrome. A prothrombotic state has been implicated in both the development of atherosclerosis[100] and the occurrence of major cardiovascular events.[101]

Patients with the metabolic syndrome have the characteristics of a prothrombotic state. They commonly have high levels of both PAI-1 and fibrinogen.[102,103] Excess adipose tissue, characteristic of people with the metabolic syndrome, has been shown to produce increased amounts of PAI-1.[92,93] Fibrinogen is an acute-phase reactant characteristic of a proinflammatory state, as discussed earlier. The literature strongly suggests that individuals with elevated concentrations of PAI-1 and fibrinogen are at increased risk for major cardiovascular events.[104-106]

Type II Diabetes
Insulin resistance as a predictor of diabetes

People with the metabolic syndrome are at increased risk for type 2 diabetes because most of them have insulin resistance. To develop categoric hyperglycemia (ie, diabetes) there must be a coexisting decrease in insulin secretion. Diabetes rarely develops in people who can respond to insulin resistance with enough newly secreted insulin. However, insulin secretory capacity typically declines with age, more rapidly in some people than in others. Slower secretors may have a genetic predisposition to loss of insulin secretion. When insulin secretion declines to the point that circulating levels cannot overcome a given level of insulin resistance, hyperglycemia develops. This sequence is the usual mechanism for development of type 2 diabetes. At least one third of people with the metabolic syndrome will develop type 2 diabetes sometime in life.[107] However, diabetes typically occurs relatively late during the course of the metabolic syndrome.[107]

A transitional state generally exists on the pathway to diabetes; this condition is called *prediabetes*. The American Diabetes Association defines prediabetes as a fasting glucose level of 100 to 126 mg/dL.[108] This level is also called *impaired fasting glucose* (IFG). Another indicator of plasma glucose abnormality on the way to diabetes is impaired glucose tolerance (IGT). IGT is defined as a 2-hour postprandial glucose level of 140 to 199 mg/dL following a 75 g OGTT. Most people with IFG/IGT can be considered to have the metabolic syndrome. In the discussion to follow, evidence relating IFG/IGT to type 2 diabetes will be reviewed. In the studies, criteria used to define IFG, IGT, and type 2 diabetes were similar, although not always identical.

The Baltimore Longitudinal Study of Aging[109] followed 285 women and 530 men with an initial mean age of 57 years for more than 10 years. Of the 60% who began with normal glucose tolerance, 14% had progressed to IFG, and

48% to IGT by 10 years. Of the 267 subjects who progressed to IFG-IGT, 216 continued follow-up. By 10 years, 8% of these progressed to diabetes by fasting hyperglycemia, whereas 27% had diabetes as shown by OGTT.

The results of these studies provide the basis for the argument that failure to carry out OGTT in higher-risk individuals will cause failure to identify many who will progress to diabetes. This could be important for the prevention of diabetes. Early detection of enhanced risk could allow for institution of more intensive prevention programs. On the other hand, the relatively slow rate of progression to diabetes from IGT raises the question of whether investment in the resources required to detect a higher risk for diabetes is cost-effective.

Many people have insulin resistance without any abnormality in glucose levels or tolerance. It is from this pool of people that most cases of IGT and IFG eventually develop. Some individuals may become glucose intolerant without insulin resistance, but they are relatively rare. Thus, insulin resistance must be considered a risk factor for type 2 diabetes.

Proinflammatory state as predictor of diabetes

Because of growing interest in a link between inflammation and metabolism, a key question is whether inflammatory processes may play a role in causing type 2 diabetes. Two general mechanisms have been proposed. First, development of insulin resistance may have an inflammatory component. Second, inflammation may play a role in loss of insulin secretory capacity by islet β-cells. Most of the evidence relating inflammation to type 2 diabetes is indirect. Nonetheless, it is of potential interest and should be reviewed.

One line of evidence for an association between inflammation and type 2 diabetes is the observation that patients with this form of diabetes commonly show elevations of either proinflammatory cytokines or acute-phase reactants. The former include interleukin-6 and TNF-α, whereas the latter are CRP, fibrinogen, and serum amyloid A (SAA).

Elevated white blood count (WBC) may also indicate low-grade inflammation.

The origins of these blood abnormalities are not fully understood. Adipose tissue itself has been reported to secrete TNF,[110] complement system products, macrophage colony-stimulating factor, and several interleukins, including IL-6. In one study, obese subjects produced 7.5 times as much TNF as lean subjects. Apparently, visceral adipose tissue produces more inflammatory chemicals than subcutaneous adipose tissue.[2,21] Although cytokine production by subcutaneous adipose tissue has been reported, it has not been adequately confirmed. Because the volume of subcutaneous adipose tissue greatly exceeds that of visceral adipose tissue, the former could produce more cytokines than the latter even if the latter were to be more active on a gram-by-gram basis.

Evidence that a proinflammatory state precedes the development of type 2 diabetes comes from prospective studies that have identified elevations of the CRP, an acute-phase reactant. Higher levels of CRP presumably reflect the presence of excess cytokines in the liver, which is the major site of CRP synthesis. Certainly a high production of CRP by the liver is responsible for the marked elevations in this protein and other acute-phase reactants associated with clinical infections and exacerbations of autoimmune disease. Some prospective data show an association between serum inflammatory markers, such as CRP, and risk for developing type 2 diabetes. In one of the three MONICA (Monitoring of Trends and Determinants in Cardiovascular Disease) surveys of 2,052 initially nondiabetic men aged 45 to 74 years followed for an average of 7.2 years, men with CRP levels in the highest quartile had a 2.7 times higher risk of developing diabetes than men in the lowest quartile.[111]

In the Insulin Resistance Atherosclerosis Study, a significant association of CRP and fibrinogen with the incidence of diabetes was reported.[103]

References

1.   Wilson P, D'Agostino RB, Sullivan L, et al: Overweight and obesity as determinants of cardiovascular risk: the Framingham experience. *Arch Intern Med* 2002;162:1867-1872.

2.   Rexrode KM, Carey VJ, Hennekens CH, et al: Abdominal adiposity and coronary heart disease in women. *JAMA* 1998;280: 1843-8148.

3.   Banegas JR, Rodriguez-Artalejo F, Graciani A, et al: Mortality attributable to cardiovascular risk factors in Spain. *Eur J Clin Nutr* 2003;57(suppl 1):S18-S21.

4.   Van Gaal LF, Wauters MA, De Leeuw IH: The beneficial effects of modest weight loss on cardiovascular risk factors. *Int J Obes Relat Metab Disord* 1997;21(suppl 1):S5-S9.

5.   Hecker KD, Kris-Etherton PM, Zhao G, et al: Impact of body weight and weight loss on cardiovascular risk factors. *Curr Atheroscler Rep* 1999;1:236-242.

6.   Krebs JD, Evans S, Cooney L, et al: Changes in risk factors for cardiovascular disease with body fat loss in obese women. *Diabetes Obes Metab* 2002;4:379-387.

7.   Miller ER 3rd, Erlinger TP, Young DR, et al: Results of the Diet, Exercise, and Weight Loss Intervention Trial (DEW-IT). *Hypertension* 2002;40:612-618.

8.   Parker B, Noakes M, Luscombe N, et al: Effect of a high-protein, high-monounsaturated fat weight loss diet on glycemic control and lipid levels in type 2 diabetes. *Diabetes Care* 2002;25: 425-340.

9.   Gaede P, Vedel P, Larsen N, et al: Multifactorial intervention and cardiovascular disease in patients with type 2 diabetes. *N Engl J Med* 2003;348:383-393.

10.   Esposito K, Pontillo A, Di Palo C, et al: Effect of weight loss and lifestyle changes on vascular inflammatory markers in obese women: a randomized trial. *JAMA* 2003;289:1799-1804.

11.   Wilson PWF, D'Agostino RB, Levy D, et al: Prediction of coronary heart disease using risk factor categories. *Circulation* 1998; 97:1837-1847.

12.   American Heart Association. Web site http://www.americanheart.org/presenter.jhtml?identifier=106. Accessed February 19, 2005.

13. *Third Report of the National Cholesterol Education Program (NCEP) Expert Panel on Detection, Evaluation, and Treatment of High Blood Cholesterol in Adults (Adult Treatment Panel III)*. US Department of Health and Human Services. National Institutes of Health. National Heart, Lung, and Blood Institute. September 2002. NIH Publication No. 02-5215.

14. US Department of Health and Human Services. Physical activity and health: a report of the Surgeon General. Atlanta, Georgia: US Department of Health and Human Services, Centers for Disease Control and Prevention, National Center for Chronic Disease Prevention and Health Promotion, 1996; 278 pages.

15. Blair SN, Haskell WL, Ho P, et al: Assessment of habitual physical activity by a seven-day recall in a community survey and controlled experiments. *Am J Epidemiol* 1985;122:794-804.

16. Imazu M: Hypertension and insulin disorders. *Curr Hypertens Rep* 2002;4:477-482.

17. Durstine JL, Grandjean PW, Cox CA, et al: Lipids, lipoproteins, and exercise. *J Cardiopulm Rehabil* 2002;22:385-398.

18. Perseghin G, Price TB, Petersen KF, et al: Increased glucose transport-phosphorylation and muscle glycogen synthesis after exercise training in insulin-resistant subjects. *N Engl J Med* 1996;335:1357-1362.

19. Henriksen EJ: Invited review: Effects of acute exercise and exercise training on insulin resistance. *J Appl Physiol* 2002;93:788-796.

20. Willey KA, Singh MA: Battling insulin resistance in elderly obese people with type 2 diabetes: bring on the heavy weights. *Diabetes Care* 2003;26:1580-1588.

21. Zierath JR: Invited review: Exercise training-induced changes in insulin signaling in skeletal muscle. *J Appl Physiol* 2002;93:773-781.

22. Sherman SE, D'Agostino RB, Silbershatz H, et al: Comparison of past versus recent physical activity in the prevention of premature death and coronary artery disease. *Am Heart J* 1999;138 (5 Pt 1):900-907.

23. Ellekjaer H, Holmen J, Ellekjaer E, et al: Physical activity and stroke mortality in women. Ten-year follow-up of the Nord-Trondelag health survey, 1984-1986. *Stroke* 2000;31:14-18.

24. Bowles DK, Wamhoff BR: Coronary smooth muscle adaptation to exercise: does it play a role in cardioprotection? *Acta Physiol Scand* 2003;178:117-121.

25.   Powers SK, Lennon SL, Quindry J, et al: Exercise and cardioprotection. *Curr Opin Cardiol* 2002;17:495-502.

26.   Kannel WB, Belanger A, D'Agostino R, et al: Physical activity and physical demand on the job and risk of cardiovascular disease and death: The Framingham Study. *Am Heart J* 1986;112:820-825.

27.   Blair SN, Shaten J, Brownell K, et al: Body weight change, all-cause mortality, and cause-specific mortality in the Multiple Risk Factor Intervention Trial. *Ann Intern Med* 1993;119(7 Pt 2): 749-757.

28.   Krauss RM, Eckel RH, Howard B, et al: AHA Dietary Guidelines: revision 2000: A statement for healthcare professionals from the Nutrition Committee of the American Heart Association. *Circulation* 2000;102:2284-2299.

29.   US Department of Agriculture and US Department of Health and Human Services. Nutrition and your health: dietary guidelines for Americans, 5th edition. Home and Garden Bulletin no. 232. Washington, DC: US Department of Agriculture, 2000;44 pages.

30.   National Institutes of Health: Clinical guidelines on the identification, evaluation, and treatment of overweight and obesity in adults—the evidence report. *Obesity Res* 1998;6(suppl 2):51S-209S.

31.   Grundy SM, Hansen B, Smith SC Jr, et al: Clinical management of metabolic syndrome: report of the American Heart Association/National Heart, Lung, and Blood Institute/American Diabetes Association conference on scientific issues related to management. *Circulation* 2004;109:551-556.

32.   Verges BL: Dyslipidaemia in diabetes mellitus: Review of the main lipoprotein abnormalities and their consequences on the development of atherogenesis. *Diabetes Metab* 1999;25(suppl 3): 32-40.

33.   Durrington PN: Diabetic dyslipidaemia. *Baillière's Clin Endocrinol Metab* 1999;13:265-278.

34.   Assmann G, Schulte H, Funke H, et al: The emergence of triglycerides as a significant independent risk factor in coronary artery disease. *Eur Heart J* 1998;19(suppl M):M8-M14.

35.   Havel RJ: Role of triglyceride-rich lipoproteins in progression of atherosclerosis. *Circulation* 1990;81:694-696.

36.   Nordestgaard BG, Lewis B: Intermediate density lipoprotein levels are strong predictors of the extent of aortic atherosclerosis in the St. Thomas's Hospital rabbit strain. *Atherosclerosis* 1991;87:39-46.

37. Breslow JL: Mouse models of atherosclerosis. *Science* 1996; 272:685-688.

38. Hodis HN, Mack WJ, Azen SP, et al: Triglyceride- and cholesterol-rich lipoproteins have a differential effect on mild/moderate and severe lesion progression as assessed by quantitative coronary angiography in a controlled trial of lovastatin. *Circulation* 1994;90:42-49.

39. Koren E, Corder C, Mueller G, et al: Triglyceride enriched lipoprotein particles correlate with the severity of coronary artery disease. *Atherosclerosis* 1996;122:105-105.

40. Karpe F, Boquist S, Tang R, et al: Remnant lipoproteins are related to intima-media thickness of the carotid artery independently of LDL cholesterol and plasma triglycerides. *J Lipid Res* 2001;42:17-21.

41. Sacks FM, Alaupovic P, Moye LA, et al: VLDL, apolipoproteins B, CIII, and E, and risk of recurrent coronary events in the Cholesterol and Recurrent Events (CARE) trial. *Circulation* 2000;102:1886-1892.

42. Vega GL, Grundy SM: Lipoprotein responses to treatment with lovastatin, gemfibrozil, and nicotinic acid in normolipidemic patients with hypoalphalipoproteinemia. *Arch Intern Med* 1994;154:73-82.

43. Martin-Jadraque R, Tato F, Mostaza JM, et al: Effectiveness of low-dose crystalline nicotinic acid in men with low high-density lipoprotein cholesterol levels. *Arch Intern Med* 1996;156:1081-1088.

44. Guyton JR, Blazing MA, Hagar J, et al: Extended-release niacin vs gemfibrozil for the treatment of low levels of high-density lipoprotein cholesterol. Niaspan-Gemfibrozil Study Group. *Arch Intern Med* 2000;160:1177-1184.

45. Zema MJ: Gemfibrozil, nicotinic acid and combination therapy in patients with isolated hypoalphalipoproteinemia: a randomized, open-label, crossover study. *J Am Coll Cardiol* 2000;35:640-646.

46. Frost PH, Havel RJ: Rationale for use of non-high-density lipoprotein cholesterol rather than low-density lipoprotein cholesterol as a tool for lipoprotein cholesterol screening and assessment of risk and therapy. *Am J Cardiol* 1998;81:26B-31B.

47. Stone NJ: Secondary causes of hyperlipidemia. *Med Clin North Am* 1994;78:117-141.

48. Chait A, Brunzell JD: Acquired hyperlipidemia (secondary dyslipoproteinemias). *Endocrinol Metab Clin North Am* 1990;19: 259-278.

49.   Denke MA, Sempos CT, Grundy SM: Excess body weight. An under-recognized contributor to dyslipidemia in white American women. *Arch Intern Med* 1994;154:401-410.

50.   Gardner CD, Fortmann SP, Krauss RM: Association of small low-density lipoprotein particles with the incidence of coronary artery disease in men and women. *JAMA* 1996;276:875-881.

51.   Gordon DJ, Probstfield JL, Garrison RJ, et al: High-density lipoprotein cholesterol and cardiovascular disease: four prospective American studies. *Circulation* 1989;79:8-15.

52.   Tall AR: An overview of reverse cholesterol transport. *Eur Heart J* 1998;19(suppl A):A31-A35.

53.   Navab M, Hama SY, Cooke CJ, et al: Normal high density lipoprotein inhibits three steps in the formation of mildly oxidized low density lipoprotein: step 1. *J Lipid Res* 2000;41:1481-1494.

54.   Schaefer EJ, Lamon-Fava S, Ordovas JM, et al: Factors associated with low and elevated plasma high density lipoprotein cholesterol and apolipoprotein A-I levels in the Framingham Offspring Study. *J Lipid Res* 1994;35:871-882.

55.   Austin MA, Rodriguez BL, McKnight B, et al: Low-density lipoprotein particle size, triglycerides, and high-density lipoprotein cholesterol as risk factors for coronary heart disease in older Japanese-American men. *Am J Cardiol* 2000;86:412-416.

56.   Cohen JC, Wang Z, Grundy SM, et al: Variation at the hepatic lipase and apolipoprotein AI/CIII/AIV loci is a major cause of genetically determined variation in plasma HDL cholesterol levels. *J Clin Invest* 1994;94:2377-2384.

57.   Brown CD, Higgins M, Donato KA, et al: Body mass index and the prevalence of hypertension and dyslipidemia. *Obes Res* 2000; 8:605-619.

58.   Bloch S, Couderc R: Apolipoprotein B and LDL cholesterol: which parameter(s) should be included in the assessment of cardiovascular risk? *Ann Biol Clin (Paris)* 1998;56:539-544.

59.   MacMahon S, Peto R, Cutler J, et al: Blood pressure, stroke, and coronary heart disease. Part 1, prolonged differences in blood pressure: prospective observational studies corrected for the regression dilution bias. *Lancet* 1990;335:765-774.

60.   Staessen JA, Fagard R, Thijs L, et al: Randomised double-blind comparison of placebo and active treatment for older persons

with isolated systolic hypertension. The Systolic Hypertension in Europe (Syst-Eur) Trial Investigators. *Lancet* 1997;1:757-764.

61. Franklin SS, Khan SA, Wong ND, et al: Is pulse pressure useful in predicting risk for coronary heart disease? The Framingham heart study. *Circulation* 1999;100:354-360.

62. van den Hoogen PC, Feskens EJ, Nagelkerke NJ, et al: The relation between blood pressure and mortality due to coronary heart disease among men in different parts of the world. Seven Countries Research Group. *N Engl J Med* 2000;342:1-8.

63. Vasan RS, Larson MG, Evans JC, et al: High normal blood pressure and risk of cardiovascular disease: the Framingham Heart Study. *Circulation* 1999;100(suppl 1):34.

64. Cutler JA, Psaty BM, MacMahon S, et al: Public health issues in hypertension control: what has been learned from clinical trials. In: Laragh JH, Brenner BM eds. *Hypertension: Pathophysiology, Diagnosis, and Management.* 2nd ed, New York: Raven Press, 1995: 253-270.

65. Sowers JR, Epstein M, Frohlich ED: Diabetes, hypertension, and cardiovascular disease: an update. *Hypertension* 2001;37:1053-1059.

66. Pyorala M, Miettinen H, Halonen P, et al: Insulin resistance syndrome predicts the risk of coronary heart disease and stroke in healthy middle-aged men: the 22-year follow-up results of the Helsinki Policemen Study. *Arterioscler Thromb Vasc Biol* 2000; 20:538-544.

67. Kuusisto J, Lempiainen P, Mykkanen L, et al: Insulin resistance syndrome predicts coronary heart disease events in elderly type 2 diabetic men. *Diabetes Care* 2001;24:1629-1633.

68. Piedrola G, Novo E, Serrano-Gotarredona J, et al: Insulin resistance in patients with a recent diagnosis of coronary artery disease. *J Hypertens* 1996;14:1477-1482.

69. Adler AI, Neil HA, Manley SE, et al: Hyperglycemia and hyperinsulinemia at diagnosis of diabetes and their association with subsequent cardiovascular disease in the United Kingdom prospective diabetes study (UKPDS 47). *Am Heart J* 1999;138(5 Pt 1): S353-S359.

70. Kamide K, Rakugi H, Nakano N, et al: Insulin resistance is related to silent cerebral infarction in patients with essential hypertension. *Am J Hypertens* 1997;10:1245-1249.

71. Reaven GM: The kidney: an unwilling accomplice in syndrome X. *Am J Kidney Dis* 1997;30:928-931.

72. Quinones-Galvan A, Ferrannini E: Renal effects of insulin in man. *J Nephrol* 1997;10:188-191.

73. Reaven GM: Pathophysiology of insulin resistance in human disease. *Physiol Rev* 1995;75:473-486.

74. Ruotolo G, Howard BV: Dyslipidemia of the metabolic syndrome. *Curr Cardiol Rep* 2002;4:494-500.

75. Corry DB, Tuck ML: Obesity, hypertension, and sympathetic nervous system activity. *Curr Hypertens Rep* 1999;1:119-126.

76. Lyon CJ, Law RE, Hsueh WA: Minireview: adiposity, inflammation, and atherogenesis. *Endocrinology* 2003;144:2195-2200.

77. Pajvani UB, Scherer PE: Adiponectin: systemic contributor to insulin sensitivity. *Curr Diab Rep* 2003;3:207-213.

78. Egan BM: Insulin resistance and the sympathetic nervous system. *Curr Hypertens Rep* 2003;5:247-254.

79. Camejo G: PPAR agonists in the treatment of insulin resistance and associated arterial disease. *Int J Clin Pract Suppl* 2003; 134:36-44.

80. Reaven GM, Mondon CE: Effect of in vivo plasma insulin levels on the relationship between perfusate free fatty acid concentration and triglyceride secretion by perfused rat livers. *Horm Metab Res* 1984;16:230-232.

81. Temelkova-Kurktschiev T, Henkel E, Schaper F, et al: Prevalence and atherosclerosis risk in different types of non-diabetic hyperglycemia. Is mild hyperglycemia an underestimated evil? *Exp Clin Endocrinol Diabetes* 2000;108:93-99.

82. Antonicelli R, Gesuita R, Boemi M, et al: Random fasting hyperglycemia as cardiovascular risk factor in the elderly: a 6-year longitudinal study. *Clin Cardiol* 2001;24:341-344.

83. Adler AI, Stevens RJ, Neil A, et al: UKPDS 59: hyperglycemia and other potentially modifiable risk factors for peripheral vascular disease in type 2 diabetes. *Diabetes Care* 2002;25:894-899.

84. Mikhail N: Postprandial hyperglycemia and risk of atherosclerosis. *JAMA* 2002;288:955.

85. Gerich JE: Clinical significance, pathogenesis, and management of postprandial hyperglycemia. *Arch Intern Med* 2003;163: 1306-1316.

86.   Schmidt AM, Yan SD, Wautier JL: Activation of receptor for advanced glycation end products: a mechanism for chronic vascular dysfunction in diabetic vasculopathy and atherosclerosis. *Circ Res* 1999;84:489-497.

87.   Gross ER, LaDisa JF Jr, Weihrauch D, et al: Reactive oxygen species modulate coronary wall shear stress and endothelial function during hyperglycemia. *Am J Physiol Heart Circ Physiol* 2003; 284:H1552-H1559.

88.   Gresele P, Guglielmini G, De Angelis M, et al: Acute, short-term hyperglycemia enhances shear stress-induced platelet activation in patients with type II diabetes mellitus. *J Am Coll Cardiol* 2003;41:1013-1020.

89.   Sampson MJ, Davies IR, Brown JC, et al: Monocyte and neutrophil adhesion molecule expression during acute hyperglycemia and after antioxidant treatment in type 2 diabetes and control patients. *Arterioscler Thromb Vasc Biol* 2002;22:1187-1193.

90.   Bruun JM, Lihn AS, Verdich C, et al: Regulation of adiponectin by adipose tissue-derived cytokines: in vivo and in vitro investigations in humans. *Am J Physiol Endocrinol Metab* 2003;285:E527-E533.

91.   Zoccali C, Mallamaci F, Tripepi G: Adipose tissue as a source of inflammatory cytokines in health and disease: focus on end-stage renal disease. *Kidney Int Suppl* 2003;84:S65-S68.

92.   Udden J, Eriksson P, Hoffstedt J: Glucocorticoid-regulated adipose tissue secretion of PAI-1, but not IL-6, TNF alpha or leptin in vivo. *Horm Metab Res* 2002;34:698-702.

93.   Fain JN, Kanu A, Bahouth SW, et al: Comparison of PGE2, prostacyclin and leptin release by human adipocytes versus explants of adipose tissue in primary culture. *Prostaglandins Leukot Essent Fatty Acids* 2002;67:467-473.

94.   Saltiel AR: New perspectives into the molecular pathogenesis and treatment of type 2 diabetes. *Cell* 2001;104:517-529.

95.   Ridker PM: High-sensitivity C-reactive protein and cardiovascular risk: rationale for screening and primary prevention. *Am J Cardiol* 2003;92:17K-22K.

96.   Abrams J: C-reactive protein, inflammation, and coronary risk: an update. *Cardiol Clin* 2003;21:327-331.

97.   Albert MA, Glynn RJ, Ridker PM: Plasma concentration of C-reactive protein and the calculated Framingham Coronary Heart Disease Risk Score. *Circulation* 2003;108:161-165.

98. Black PH: The inflammatory response is an integral part of the stress response: Implications for atherosclerosis, insulin resistance, type II diabetes and metabolic syndrome X. *Brain Behav Immun* 2003;17:350-364.

99. Mertens I, Van Gaal LF: Obesity, haemostasis and the fibrinolytic system. *Obes Rev* 2002;3:85-101.

100. Juhan-Vague I, Alessi MC: Regulation of fibrinolysis in the development of atherothrombosis: role of adipose tissue. *Thromb Haemost* 1999;82:832-836.

101. Niessner A, Graf S, Nikfardjam M, et al: Circulating t-PA antigen predicts major adverse coronary events in patients with stable coronary artery disease—a 13-year follow-up. *Thromb Haemost* 2003;90:344-350.

102. Decsi T, Molnar D: Insulin resistance syndrome in children: pathophysiology and potential management strategies. *Paediatr Drugs* 2003;5:291-299.

103. Festa A, D'Agostino R Jr, Tracy RP, et al: Elevated levels of acute-phase proteins and plasminogen activator inhibitor-1 predict the development of type 2 diabetes: the insulin resistance atherosclerosis study. *Diabetes* 2002;51:1131-1137.

104. Haverkate F: Levels of haemostatic factors, arteriosclerosis and cardiovascular disease. *Vascul Pharmacol* 2002;39:109-112.

105. Junker R, Heinrich J, Schulte H, et al: Hemostasis in normotensive and hypertensive men: results of the PROCAM study. The prospective cardiovascular Munster study. *J Hypertens* 1998;16:917-923.

106. Folsom AR, Pankow JS, Williams RR, et al: Fibrinogen, plasminogen activator inhibitor-1, and carotid intima-media wall thickness in the NHLBI Family Heart Study. *Thromb Haemost* 1998;79:400-404.

107. Sattar N, Gaw A, Scherbakova O, et al. Metabolic syndrome with and without C-reactive protein as a predictor of coronary heart disease and diabetes in the West of Scotland Coronary Prevention Study. *Circulation* 2003;108:414-419.

108. Benjamin SM, Valdez R, Geiss LS, et al: Estimated number of adults with prediabetes in the US in 2000: opportunities for prevention. *Diabetes Care* 2003;26:645-649.

109. Meigs JB, Muller DC, Nathan DM, et al: The natural history of progression from normal glucose tolerance to type 2 diabetes in

the Baltimore Longitudinal Study of Aging. *Diabetes* 2003;52: 1475-1484.

110. Kern PA, Ranganathan S, Li C, et al: Adipose tissue tumor necrosis factor and interleukin-6 expression in human obesity and insulin resistance. *Am J Physiol Endocrinol Metab* 2001;280:E745-E751.

111. Thorand B, Lowel H, Schneider A, et al: C-reactive protein as a predictor for incident diabetes mellitus among middle-aged men: results from the MONICA Augsburg cohort study, 1984-1998. *Arch Intern Med* 2003;163:93-99.

Chapter 6

Clinical Assessment and Diagnosis of the Metabolic Syndrome

Although the concept of the metabolic syndrome has existed in various forms for many years, clinical criteria for its diagnosis were not formalized in a way that was useful in clinical practice. Thus, for a long time, the syndrome was recognized by clinical research and pathophysiology, but was not routinely identified in patients.

Recently, however, attempts have been made to define the criteria that permit a clinical diagnosis of the metabolic syndrome. In 1998 and 1999, a World Health Organization (WHO) committee on diabetes outlined the clinical characteristics required for a diagnosis of the metabolic syndrome.[1,2] These criteria were not widely disseminated to the medical community and thus were sparsely applied. More recently, the National Cholesterol Education Program's Adult Treatment Panel III (NCEP ATP III) proposed a somewhat different list of criteria.[3] Because these criteria were linked to widely used clinical guidelines for cholesterol management, they received greater attention. Although ATP III undoubtedly gave the concept a boost, the recommendations were well received because of the increasing prevalence of the metabolic syndrome in the United States. Other criteria for the metabolic syndrome have been proposed and will also be considered in this chapter.

It is important to differentiate between the definition of the metabolic syndrome and the clinical criteria required for diagnosis. The two are not necessarily the same, and failure to make a distinction has led to confusion. Chapter 1 deals with definition; this chapter will focus on clinical criteria for diagnosis.

Because the metabolic syndrome is complex, diagnostic criteria must attempt to capture the essence of the condition without necessarily incorporating all of the components. Clinical criteria must also be applicable in daily practice. One limitation of some of the criteria is that they require special testing beyond what is available in routine practice. Special testing may provide additional useful information, but it adds expense and inconvenience that reduce its usefulness in practice.

Research groups, the pharmaceutical industry, and regulatory agencies have expressed interest in criteria for clinical diagnosis of the metabolic syndrome. These groups would like a 'consensus' definition that can be universally used. This chapter attempts to develop diagnosis criteria that are useful in routine clinical practice.

ATP III Clinical Criteria

Metabolic Syndrome as a Secondary Target of Therapy in Cholesterol Treatment Guidelines

A primary goal of the NCEP has been to develop evidence-based recommendations for clinical management of high blood cholesterol levels in adults. To date, three Adult Treatment Panel (ATP) reports have been released, the first (ATP I) in 1988.[4] ATP I's justification for advocating cholesterol management was based on epidemiologic evidence, animal studies, limited clinical trial data, and genetic forms of hypercholesterolemia, including genetic disorders of low-density lipoprotein (LDL) metabolism such as familial hypercholesterolemia and polygenic hypercholesterolemia that frequently manifest premature atherosclerotic disease even without other risk factors. Other clinical evidence for cholesterol management included large epidemiologic surveys that had identified a relationship between serum total cholesterol and risk for coronary heart disease (CHD).[5-8] In 1984,[9,10] the Lipid Research Clinic (LRC) Coronary Primary Prevention Trial (CPPT) compared a cholesterol-lowering drug, cholestyramine, to placebo for efficacy in patients with primary hypercholesterolemia. The result was positive for major coronary events. Cholestyramine therapy reduced the primary end point, CHD events, and coronary death. This combined evidence was considered sufficient to warrant inclusion in the NCEP.

Because most of the evidence pointed to LDL cholesterol (LDL-C) as the major atherogenic lipoprotein, ATP I identified LDL-C as the primary target of lipid-lowering therapy. That LDL-C should be the first and major target of therapy was supported in subsequent ATP reports.

In 1993, ATP II retained strong support for LDL lowering through dietary means for primary prevention of CHD. Moreover, a meta-analysis of secondary prevention trials of cholesterol-lowering therapy[11-14] indicated that reducing serum cholesterol was effective in preventing major coronary events and coronary death. The ATP II panel therefore emphasized cholesterol-lowering therapy in patients with established CHD (secondary prevention). Indeed, the panel recommended that LDL-C be reduced to <100 mg/dL in patients with established CHD. ATP II also recommended increased emphasis on obesity and physical inactivity as secondary targets of lipid-lowering therapy. The goal was twofold: (1) to achieve enhanced LDL reduction and (2) to improve other lipid risk factors (ie, low HDL-C and high triglyceride levels). This recommendation was based on growing evidence that low HDL and high triglyceride levels carried atherogenic potential beyond elevated LDL-C.

In 2001, ATP III strengthened the case for LDL-lowering therapy in primary and secondary prevention, based on clinical trials with HMG CoA reductase inhibitors (statins) that showed marked reductions in risk for CHD. Because effective statin therapy was available, recommendations for intensive treatment of LDL-C with drugs were greatly expanded. ATP III emphasized identifying an individual's risk category (Table 6-1). The concept of secondary prevention was extended to high-risk prevention. Patients at high risk have either established CHD or conditions called *CHD risk equivalents*. In other words, if a person without established CHD has a risk for future major coronary events equal to that of someone with CHD, this person is said to have a CHD risk equivalent. Included in this category are patients with clinical forms of atherosclerotic disease (eg, peripheral arterial disease, abdominal aortic aneurysm, and carotid artery disease), patients with diabetes, and those with multiple factors that raise the risk for major coronary events (myocardial infarction + coronary death) to >20% in 10 years. Evidence indicates that a person with established CHD has a 10-year risk of at least 20% for major coronary events. For high-risk patients (ie, those with CHD or CHD risk equivalents), an LDL-C goal of <100 mg/dL was established.

ATP III further recognized a risk category called *moderately high risk*, defined as two or more major risk factors plus a 10-year risk for major coronary events of 10% to 20%. The major risk factors other than elevated LDL-C include cigarette smoking; hypertension (blood pressure >140/90 mm Hg or on treatment for hypertension); low HDL cholesterol (HDL-C) (<40 mg/dL); family history of premature CHD in first-degree relative (men <55 years; women <60 years); and advancing age (men >45 years; women >55 years). Diabetes is a major risk factor for CHD, but its presence, in most patients, equates to a CHD risk equivalent.

In ATP III, the 10-year risk for CHD specifies myocardial infarction or coronary death. Estimation of 10-

Table 6-1: Risk Categories of Adult Treatment Panel III Report

Risk Category	Features of Risk Category

High risk	Established coronary heart disease
	   - peripheral arterial disease
	   - abdominal aortic aneurysm
	   - clinical carotid artery disease
	   - diabetes
	
	2+ major risk factors* and 10-year risk for CHD >20%**

Moderately high risk	2+ major risk factors* and 10-year risk for CHD 10%-20%
Moderate risk	2+ major risk factors* and 10-year risk for CHD <10%**
Lower risk	0-1 risk factor* or 10-year risk for CHD <10%**

* Major risk factors include cigarette smoking, hypertension (blood pressure >140/90 mm Hg or on treatment for hypertension), low HDL cholesterol (<40 mg/dL), family history of premature CHD in first-degree relative (men <55 years; women <60 years), and advancing age (men >45 years; women >55 years).

** 10-year risk for CHD determined by Framingham risk algorithm (see Tables 6-2 and 6-3).

CHD = coronary heart disease

year risk for CHD is made with the Framingham Study risk algorithm. Factors included in this algorithm are cigarette smoking, total cholesterol, HDL-C, blood pressure, and age.

Estimates of 10-year risk can be obtained from Table 6-2 and Table 6-3 or by computer program. Computer assessment of risk can be obtained online at www.nhlbi.nih.gov under Cholesterol Guidelines.

For persons who have two or more risk factors plus a 10-year risk <10% (moderate risk), the treatment goal for LDL-C is still <130 mg/dL, but drug therapy guidelines are less strict. Most persons with 0-1 risk factor (lower risk) have a 10-year risk <10%. Therefore, Framingham risk scoring is not necessary. The LDL-C goal for those with 0-1 risk factor is <160 mg/dL.

Introduction of the Metabolic Syndrome
Into ATP III Guidelines

The 1993 ATP II report recognized the high prevalence of obesity and physical inactivity in the United States. It placed increased emphasis on weight reduction in overweight/obese persons and increased physical activity in sedentary individuals. Unfortunately, these recommendations had little impact on the cardiovascular community. Therefore, ATP III considered methods to focus attention on obesity and physical inactivity. It identified the metabolic syndrome as a major, complex risk factor that results largely from obesity and sedentary life habits. The ATP III treatment algorithm focused on managing of high LDL-C, but once the goals of LDL lowering were attained, attention shifted to the metabolic syndrome and its risk factors. It is important to note that the metabolic syndrome does not include elevated LDL-C, although the two conditions may coexist. For management of the metabolic syndrome, modification of its underlying causes, (ie, overweight/obesity and physical inactivity) took priority.

ATP III Criteria for Clinical Diagnosis
of the Metabolic Syndrome

The introduction of specific criteria for clinical diagnosis of the metabolic syndrome gives the health profession a way to identify patients at increased risk for both atherosclerotic cardiovascular disease (ASCVD) and type 2 dia-

Table 6-2: Framingham Point Scores Estimate of 10-Year Risk for Men

Age, years	Points
20-34	-9
35-39	-4
40-44	0
45-49	3
50-54	6
55-59	8
60-64	10
65-69	11
70-74	12
75-79	13

Total cholesterol, mg/dL	Points				
	Age 20-39y	*Age 40-49y*	*Age 50-59y*	*Age 60-69y*	*Age 70-79y*
<160	0	0	0	0	0
160-199	4	3	2	1	0
200-239	7	5	3	1	0
240-279	9	6	4	2	1
≥280	11	8	5	3	1

	Points				
	Age 20-39y	*Age 40-49y*	*Age 50-59y*	*Age 60-69y*	*Age 70-79y*
Nonsmoker	0	0	0	0	0
Smoker	8	5	3	1	1

HDL-C, mg/dL	Points
≥60	-1
50-59	0
40-49	1
<40	2

Systolic BP, mm Hg	If untreated	If treated
<120	0	0
120-129	0	1
130-139	1	2
140-159	1	2
≥160	2	3

Point total	10-year risk (%)
<0	<1
0	1
1	1
2	1
3	1
4	1
5	2
6	2
7	3
8	4
9	5
10	6
11	8
12	10
13	12
14	16
15	20
16	25
≥17	≥30

Table 6-3: Framingham Point Scores Estimate of 10-Year Risk for Women

Age, years	Points
20-34	-7
35-39	-3
40-44	0
45-49	3
50-54	6
55-59	8
60-64	10
65-69	12
70-74	14
75-79	16

Total cholesterol, mg/dL	Points				
	Age 20-39y	*Age 40-49y*	*Age 50-59y*	*Age 60-69y*	*Age 70-79y*
<160	0	0	0	0	0
160-199	4	3	2	1	1
200-239	8	6	4	2	1
240-279	11	8	5	3	2
≥280	13	10	7	4	2

	Points				
	Age 20-39y	*Age 40-49y*	*Age 50-59y*	*Age 60-69y*	*Age 70-79y*
Nonsmoker	0	0	0	0	0
Smoker	9	7	4	2	1

HDL-C, mg/dL	Points
≥60	-1
50-59	0
40-49	1
<40	2

Systolic BP, mm Hg	If untreated	If treated
<120	0	0
120-129	1	3
130-139	2	4
140-159	3	5
≥160	4	6

Point total	10-year risk (%)
<9	<1
9	1
10	1
11	1
12	1
13	2
14	2
15	3
16	4
17	5
18	6
19	8
20	11
21	14
22	17
23	22
24	27
≥25	≥30

Table 6-4: ATP III Clinical Identification of the Metabolic Syndrome

A. Risk Factor	B. Defining Level
Abdominal obesity*	Waist circumference**
Men	>102 cm (>40 in)
Women	>88 cm (>35 in)
Triglycerides	≥150 mg/dL
HDL cholesterol	
Men	<40 mg/dL
Women	<50 mg/dL
Blood pressure	≥130/≥85 mm Hg
Fasting glucose	>100 mg/dL***

* Overweight and obesity are associated with insulin resistance and the metabolic syndrome. However, abdominal obesity is more highly correlated with the metabolic risk factors than is an elevated BMI. Therefore, the simple measure of waist circumference is recommended to identify the body weight component of the metabolic syndrome.

** Some male patients, notably Asians, can develop multiple metabolic risk factors when their waist circumference is only marginally increased, eg, 94-102 cm (37-39 in). Such patients may have a strong genetic inclination to insulin resistance. They should benefit from changes in life habits similarly to men with categoric increases in waist circumference.

*** The American Diabetes Association recently redefined the lower cut point for impaired fasting glucose to be >100 mg/dL.[15]

BMI = body mass index

betes. According to ATP III, patients have the metabolic syndrome if they have three of the five characteristics shown in Table 6-4: qualifying waist circumference (surrogate for abdominal obesity), serum triglyceride levels, HDL cholesterol levels, blood pressure, and plasma glucose. Because each risk factor is a continuous variable, the cut points for each are arbitrary but appear to be typical of patients exhibiting the clustering of metabolic risk factors. Also, because any combination of three of five metabolic risk factors constitutes a diagnosis, risk factor patterns will vary from person to person. It is important to differentiate between the definition of the metabolic syndrome and the clinical criteria for diagnosis. The defining components of the metabolic syndrome are listed in Table 1-1.

ATP III diagnostic criteria for the metabolic syndrome can be easily identified in clinical practice or in epidemiologic studies, which is a major advantage. ATP III criteria do not capture all features of the syndrome, although growing evidence indicates that most individuals who exhibit the metabolic syndrome according to the ATP III criteria will have most of these features. For example, most patients with the ATP III diagnosis will be insulin resistant, even though direct measurements of their insulin sensitivity have not been done. Let us review the rationale for each characteristic of the ATP III criteria.

Rationale for ATP III Metabolic Syndrome Diagnostic Criteria

Waist Circumference

Cut points for waist circumference of >102 cm for men and >88 cm for women define abdominal obesity. These cut points were previously established by the National Institutes of Health clinical guidelines on obesity management.[16] ATP III identified obesity, particularly abdominal obesity, as a driving force of the metabolic syndrome. The increase in the metabolic syndrome in the United States is believed to be strongly associated with increasing obesity in the population.

There has been some dispute about whether whole-body obesity (indicated by elevated body mass index [BMI]) or abdominal obesity (indicated by increased waist circumference) is the better obesity-related component of the syndrome. Much evidence supports waist circumference. One rationale for use of waist circumference is shown in Table 6-4. There is considerable overlap of abdominal obesity with the categories of BMI (normal, overweight, and obesity). Most obese persons (BMI >30 kg/m^2) will have increased waist circumference, and many overweight people (BMI 25 to 30 kg/m^2) will also be abdominally obese. In fact, a small percentage of individuals with normal weight by BMI will nonetheless be abdominally obese. If BMI alone is used to identify persons in the syndrome category, the clinician will miss many with abdominal obesity.

The arbitrary cut points for abdominal obesity occur in one fourth to one third of the US population. Some authorities have suggested that lower cut points should be used as defining characteristics of the metabolic syndrome.[17] In fact, ATP III designates >94 cm as an optional increased waist circumference value for American men. In other regions of the world, lesser degrees of abdominal obesity are associated with insulin resistance and increased risk for type 2 diabetes.[18-22]

Abdominal obesity as an indicator of insulin resistance can be measured in several ways. ATP III did not recommend the commonly used waist:hip ratio. Although persons with a high waist:hip ratio frequently have insulin resistance, NIH obesity guidelines[16] judged waist circumference to be more strongly correlated with metabolic risk factors.

Elevated Triglycerides

Desirable serum levels for triglycerides are <100 mg/dL. Levels ≥150 mg/dL are commonly associated with other metabolic risk factors. ATP III defined a serum triglyceride level of 150 to 199 mg/dL as borderline high.

For most people, serum triglyceride levels in this range indicate overweight/obesity, especially abdominal obesity. Such levels point to the need for weight reduction and increased physical activity.

Reduced HDL Cholesterol

Serum HDL cholesterol levels that are lower than the mean for the population indicate metabolic abnormalities, as do elevated triglyceride levels. Thus, a reduction in HDL cholesterol can be considered a marker for the metabolic syndrome. ATP III defined reduced HDL cholesterol levels as <40 mg/dL for men and <50 mg/dL for women. As indicated earlier, a lower HDL level may directly promote atherosclerosis and is frequently associated with atherogenic dyslipidemia and other risk factors of the metabolic syndrome.

Elevated Blood Pressure

Both obesity and physical inactivity contribute to higher blood pressure. Often, the increase is relatively small, but in general, overweight/obese persons have higher blood pressures than do people of normal weight. A recent study from the Framingham Heart group[23,24] revealed that people with high-normal blood pressures (130 to 139/85 to 89 mm Hg) are at increased risk for major cardiovascular events compared to those with blood pressures <120/80 mm Hg. Therefore, ATP III set a level of ≥130/85 mm Hg as the threshold for defining the blood pressure level characteristic of the metabolic syndrome.

Recently, the Seventh Report of the Joint National Committee on Prevention, Detection, Evaluation and Treatment of High Blood Pressure (JNC 7)[25] added a new blood-pressure category—prehypertension (a blood pressure of 120 to 139/80 to 89 mm Hg). The authors of the JNC 7 report predict that most people will develop categoric hypertension (blood pressure >140/90 mm Hg) sometime in life. Persons with blood pressures in the 120 to 139/80 to 89 mm Hg range need to adopt lifestyle changes to prevent progression to categoric hypertension. For now, the ATP III threshold of 130/85 mm Hg to define the blood pressure component of the clinical metabolic syndrome still holds. The Framingham study warning about the increased risk of high-normal blood pressure provides strong evidence for ATP III's definition. A rationale for including prehypertension as the defining characteristic has not been developed.

Elevated Plasma Glucose

Most, but not all, individuals with elevated plasma glucose levels have insulin resistance as well as other features of the metabolic syndrome. Certainly, people with type 1 diabetes might not have insulin resistance, and glucose intolerance can develop in thin, elderly persons without associated insulin resistance. In other words, if pancreatic β-cell function declines enough, hyperglycemia can develop without insulin resistance. Still, most people with higher glucose levels are insulin resistant. This fact justified adding elevated plasma glucose levels to the ATP III criteria for the metabolic syndrome. Insulin resistance was not included, fundamental as it is, only because it is too difficult to measure.

The threshold level for elevated fasting glucose was set at >110 mg/dL. When the ATP III guidelines were released, the American Diabetes Association (ADA) defined impaired fasting glucose (IFG) as 110 to 125 mg/dL, and diabetes mellitus as a fasting level of >126 mg/dL.[26] The ATP III definition includes either IFG or diabetes as a defining characteristic. Thus, patients not frankly diabetic but with IFG can have the metabolic syndrome if they have two other metabolic risk factors.

After ATP III was published, the ADA lowered the threshold for elevated glucose to >100 mg/dL[15] (IFG was redefined as 100 to 125 mg/dL). This change is likely to be widely accepted as a criterion for the metabolic syndrome. If it is, more people will be identified as having the metabolic syndrome.

The ATP III definition does not include impaired glucose tolerance (IGT) (a 2-hour level >140 mg/dL following a 75 g oral glucose load). Although oral glucose tolerance testing (OGTT) would identify more persons with impaired glucose metabolism, ATP III considered such testing impractical and too expensive for routine clinical evaluation. Other authorities disagree, contending that an oral glucose challenge should be part of testing for the metabolic syndrome. The rationale for this testing will be presented later in this chapter.

Hidden Metabolic Risk Factors

The metabolic syndrome has characteristics not identified in ATP III's clinical diagnosis. They include increases in small LDL particles; elevated apolipoprotein B; hyperinsulinemia; insulin resistance by glucose-clamp study; high-normal levels of C-reactive protein (CRP); elevations of fibrinogen and PAI-I; and microalbuminuria. Research studies have shown that by ATP III definition, many of these characteristics will exist in patients who have the metabolic syndrome. Some authorities recommend that some of these measurements be included in evaluation of patients for the metabolic syndrome. While these measurements may provide incremental information about a given patient's metabolic status, they were omitted from the ATP III definition because many of them will be present in persons who carry the ATP III diagnosis, making testing for them redundant. Also, they require nonroutine testing, which can be expensive and impractical. The ATP III panel considered the simplicity of its criteria a major advantage in defining the metabolic syndrome in routine clinical practice.

World Health Organization Clinical Criteria

In 1998,[1] a WHO consultation group on diabetes classification proposed working criteria for the metabolic syndrome. Table 6-5 summarizes the WHO's 1999 modified proposal, which is available on the WHO Web site.[27]

Table 6-5: World Health Organization Clinical Criteria for Metabolic Syndrome*

Insulin resistance, identified by one of the following:

- Type 2 diabetes, impaired fasting glucose
- Impaired glucose tolerance
- For those with normal fasting glucose levels (<110 mg/dL), glucose uptake below the lowest quartile for background population under hyperinsulinemic, euglycemic conditions.

Plus any two of the following:

- Antihypertensive medication and/or high blood pressure (≥140 mm Hg systolic or ≥90 mm Hg diastolic)
- Plasma triglycerides ≥150 mg/dL (≥1.7 mmol/L)
- HDL cholesterol <35 mg/dL (<0.9 mmol/L) in men or <39 mg/dL (1.0 mmol/L) in women
- BMI >30 kg/m² and/or waist:hip ratio >0.9 in men, >0.85 in women
- Urinary albumin excretion rate ≥20 μg/min or albumin:creatinine ratio ≥30 mg/g

* World Health Organization: Definition, diagnosis and classification of diabetes mellitus and its complications: Report of a WHO Consultation. Part 1. Diagnosis and classification of diabetes mellitus. Geneva, World Health Organization, 1999 http://whqlibdoc.who.int/hq/1999/WHO_NCD_NCS_99.2.pdf.

HDL = high-density lipoprotein
BMI = body mass index

Cardiovascular disease (CVD) is recognized as the primary clinical outcome. A key feature of the WHO metabolic syndrome definition is that insulin resistance is a required constituent.

Acceptable evidence for the metabolic syndrome is one of the following: type 2 diabetes, IFG, IGT, or, for those with normal fasting glucose values (<110 mg/dL), a glucose uptake lower than the lowest quartile for the background population under hyperinsulinemic, euglycemic conditions. Two other risk factors, besides insulin resistance, are sufficient for a diagnosis.

Insulin Resistance

Evidence of insulin resistance is required for the WHO definition because many investigators believe that insulin resistance is at the core of the metabolic syndrome. This idea has been extensively developed by Reaven and associates[28-31] and others.[32-34] They hypothesize that insulin resistance might induce other metabolic risk factors. In fact, an alternate term for the metabolic syndrome is the *insulin resistance syndrome*. According to this hypothesis, obesity is only one cause of insulin resistance. Furthermore, most of the adverse metabolic effects of obesity are thought to be mediated through insulin resistance. This idea differs from that put forth in the ATP III definition, in which insulin resistance is a component of the metabolic syndrome and obesity is the driving force behind the syndrome.

According to diabetes authorities, the hyperinsulinemic-euglycemic clamp method is the gold standard for determining insulin resistance. However, this method is impractical in clinical practice. Therefore, other means of evidence are recognized as surrogate markers for insulin resistance, including type 2 diabetes, IFG, and IGT. Most people with one of these abnormalities would exhibit insulin resistance if tested by a glucose-clamp study. An alternative method for detecting insulin resistance is the HOMA measurement, calculated from the glucose/

fasting-insulin ratio.[35,36] This method was not recommended by the WHO working group but is widely recognized as an indicator of insulin sensitivity.

Although the WHO description requires evidence of insulin resistance, it is not entirely clear that this definition identifies more individuals with insulin resistance than do the ATP III criteria. All components of the ATP III definition are associated with insulin resistance, and, when at least three are present, most persons will show insulin resistance. Although WHO lists glucose-clamp studies as one way to identify insulin resistance, it admits these are impractical in clinical practice. Hyperglycemia often occurs in persons with insulin resistance, but it is as much a reflection of decline in insulin secretion as of insulin resistance. Certainly, glucose tolerance testing will improve prediction of type 2 diabetes, but WHO criteria are not likely to enhance prediction of CVD over those of ATP III.

Elevated Blood Pressure

WHO criteria, like those of ATP III, include elevated blood pressure. WHO explicitly lists antihypertensive medication as treatment. ATP III left this indicator out of its list, seemingly inadvertently. The WHO's defining level of blood pressure is higher than that of ATP III. The WHO chose the cut point for categoric hypertension ($\geq$140/90 mm Hg), while ATP III recognized high-normal blood pressure ($\geq$130/85 mm Hg). The rationale for the lower level in ATP III was stated earlier.

Elevated Plasma Triglyceride Levels

The WHO criterion for triglycerides is the same as that of ATP III (ie, levels $\geq$150 mg/dL). The rationale is also the same.

Reduced HDL Levels

The WHO panel sets lower cut points than does ATP III to define a reduced HDL-C level. For men, the level is <35 mg/dL. ATP III set a higher cut point (<40 mg/dL) because reduction of HDL-C due to obesity in the general male population rarely produces levels as low as 35 mg/dL. When HDL-C levels in men fall below 35 mg/dL, a strong genetic component usually exists. The same is true for women who meet the WHO HDL-C criteria of <39 mg/dL. The ATP III cut point of <50 mg/dL for women represents the 'metabolic' component of lower HDL without the genetic component.

Body Weight

The WHO offered two criteria for body weight indicators: BMI >30 kg/m^2 and waist:hip ratio 0.9 in men and >0.85 in women. In ATP III, BMI was rejected in favor of waist circumference, an indicator of abdominal obesity, for reasons discussed earlier. Adding the waist:hip ratio is an attempt to include a component of abdominal obesity in the WHO definition. However, most authorities believe that waist circumference is a better indicator of abdominal obesity than is the waist:hip ratio.[16]

Urinary Albumin Level

Urinary microalbuminuria is included in WHO criteria of the metabolic syndrome, for reasons not immediately evident. Microalbuminuria without diabetes presumably indicates 'vascular injury,' which might be considered a consequence of metabolic risk factors. If so, it belongs in an entirely different category of components than the other metabolic risk factors.

In summary, the WHO clinical criteria for the metabolic syndrome can be considered a precursor to the ATP III criteria. The latter contains many of the features of the former, but the ATP III definition has been updated with a broader review of the literature and a simplification that allows it to be used more readily in clinical practice without the need for special testing. Although the WHO criteria require direct evidence of insulin resistance, most people with ATP III metabolic syndrome will be insulin resistant. Also, not everyone with IFG or IGT, part of the WHO's criteria for metabolic syndrome, will be insulin resistant.

Table 6-6: European Group for the Study of Insulin Resistance

Insulin resistance: upper quartile for fasting insulin level

Plus two of the following:

- Hyperglycemia (fasting glucose >6.1 mmol/L)
- Blood pressure >140/90 mm Hg
- Serum triglyceride level >2 mmol/L
- HDL cholesterol level <1 mmol/L
- Abdominal obesity: waist circumference for men >94 cm, women >80 cm

European Group for the Study of Insulin Resistance (EGIR)

Authors for the European Group for the Study of Insulin Resistance[17] suggested a modification of WHO criteria for the metabolic syndrome. These criteria are shown in Table 6-6. Insulin resistance was retained as a requirement for the metabolic syndrome and was defined simply as a fasting insulin level in the upper quartile for the population. Other criteria include hyperglycemia, elevated blood pressure, elevated triglyceride levels (and/or reduced HDL-C), and abdominal obesity. The study set a lower cut point for elevated waist circumference (ie, >94 cm in men and >80 cm in women). These criteria have the advantage of simplicity, except for the measurement of fasting insulin. To date, accurate and standardized measurements of fasting insulin are not widely available. Even if they were available, they would be relatively expensive and not routine. Finally, it is not clear that single measurements of fasting insulin levels are a robust surrogate for insulin resistance.

American Association of Clinical Endocrinologists (AACE) Clinical Criteria

The AACE recently offered alternative clinical criteria and a different name for the metabolic syndrome: insulin resistance syndrome.[37] Most investigators equate the metabolic syndrome and the insulin resistance syndrome. However, differences in concept contribute to differences in names. The term *insulin resistance syndrome* signifies the conviction that insulin resistance is the mediating force for all metabolic risk factors. But it further means that insulin resistance is responsible for medical complications beyond the cardiovascular risk factors of the metabolic syndrome. The components of the AACE criteria are shown in Table 6-7. According to the AACE guidelines, a clinical diagnosis of the insulin resistance syndrome should be based on clinical judgment, and no specified number of risk factors is required to trigger the diagnosis.

The AACE guidelines propose a lower cut point for body weight than that used in the WHO criteria. A BMI of >25 kg/m^2 includes the categories of both overweight and obesity instead of obesity alone, as in the WHO criteria. The AACE rejected waist circumference, presumably because the recommending committee believed that a lower BMI cut point will be more inclusive of people with excess body weight than waist circumference. In other words, only some overweight people (BMI 25 to 30 kg/m^2) will have abdominal obesity as defined by ATP III. Indeed, it has been estimated that 75% of the adult population in the United States will have a BMI >25 kg/m^2. Hence, most people will have at least one AACE risk factor for the insulin resistance syndrome. The AACE adopted the same criteria as ATP III for elevation of triglyceride levels, reduction of HDL cholesterol levels, and elevation of blood pressure.

The AACE guidelines include IFG (fasting glucose 110-126 mg/dL) and IGT (2-hour postglucose challenge

Table 6-7: American Association of Clinical Endocrinologists Clinical Criteria for Diagnosis of the Insulin Resistance Syndrome*

Risk factor components	Cut points for abnormality
Overweight/obesity	BMI >25 kg/m^2
Triglycerides	≥150 mg/dL
Low HDL cholesterol	<40 mg/dL in men <50 mg/dL in women
Elevated blood pressure	≥130/85 mm Hg
2-hour postglucose challenge	>140 mg/dL
Fasting glucose	Between 110 mg/dL and 126 mg/dL
Other risk factors	Family history of type 2 diabetes, hypertension, or CVD Polycystic ovary syndrome Sedentary lifestyle Advancing age Ethnic groups having high risk for type 2 diabetes or CVD

* Diagnosis depends on clinical judgment based on risk factors.

CVD = cardiovascular disease

>140 mg/dL). By addition of the latter, the AACE is consistent with WHO criteria, but not with ATP III. As stated earlier, ATP III did not include an OGTT because of inconvenience and expense in clinical practice. Furthermore, IGT without IFG was considered by ATP III to provide neither incremental information in predicting CVD risk nor guidance for intervention to reduce this risk. According to NHANES III data,[38] if IGT were to be added to criteria for the diagnosis of the metabolic syndrome, approximately 5% of people older than 50 years would qualify.[39,40] The addition of OGTT by AACE and WHO seemingly is based on two considerations. First, IGT strongly suggests insulin resistance. Second, IGT without IFG denotes a greater risk for diabetes. Both AACE and WHO committees are diabetes-oriented groups. To them, the connection between insulin resistance and development of type 2 diabetes is critically important. The issue of OGTT points out differences in concept of the meaning of the metabolic syndrome (or the insulin resistance syndrome). ATP III focuses mainly on CVD as an outcome of metabolic syndrome, while the WHO and AACE committees shift the priority to predicting type 2 diabetes.

Because the ADA recently reduced the cut point for IFG to 100 mg/dL, fewer people will be found to have IGT without IFG. This could reduce the need for carrying out OGTT. In the diabetes field there is considerable disagreement about when to implement OGTT to identify persons at risk for type 2 diabetes. Both WHO and AACE committees support OGTT in subjects with other characteristics of the metabolic syndrome. Other criteria have been suggested by diabetes authorities: a high index of clinical suspicion, advancing age, family history of diabetes, and gestational diabetes in the past.[41]

An important point about the AACE criteria for the insulin resistance syndrome is that once categoric hyperglycemia (type 2 diabetes) intervenes, the diagnosis no longer pertains. One way to view this exclusion is that the insulin resistance syndrome is a risk factor for type 2 diabetes; type 2 diabetes is not a component of the insulin resistance syndrome. This concept differs from that held in both the ATP III and WHO criteria. The latter believe that patients with type 2 diabetes can have the metabolic syndrome if other diagnostic characteristics are present (Tables 6-4 and 6-5).

Other Features of AACE Insulin Resistance Syndrome

AACE identified these other components of insulin resistance: a family history of type 2 diabetes, hypertension, or CVD; polycystic ovary syndrome; sedentary lifestyle; advancing age; and ethnic groups with high risk for type 2 diabetes. These features are not always accompanied by insulin resistance, but they might be considered risk factors for insulin resistance. Because the AACE diagnosis of the insulin resistance syndrome does not require a specific number of risk factors, these other features can be considered modifiers that can play a role in the clinician's judgment about a given patient.

Quebec Heart Institute Hypertriglyceridemic Waist

Investigators at the Quebec Heart Institute[42-44] coined the term *hypertriglyceridemic waist* to indicate a condition with a high risk for ASCVD. This condition has many of the characteristics of the metabolic syndrome. The essential features of hypertriglyceridemic waist are an elevated waist circumference (90 cm or greater) and moderate hypertriglyceridemia (triglyceride concentration 2.0 mmol/L or higher in men). Waist measurements for women have not been specified. Other common features of the condition include a triad of metabolic markers (high insulin and apolipoprotein B levels, and small, dense, LDL particles) and a substantially increased risk of ASCVD. Men with hypertriglyceridemic waist have higher total cholesterol:HDL cholesterol ratios, which have been independently associated with insulin resistance.[44] When individuals with hypertriglyceridemic waist also have IFG, their risk for ASCVD is increased even more.[44] To date, a systematic comparison of hypertriglyceridemic waist with other clinical definitions of the metabolic syndrome (or the insulin resistance syndrome) has not been made. However, considerable overlap probably will exist. Moreover, the relationship of hypertriglyceridemic waist to the incidence (or prevalence) of ASCVD has not been made in populations outside of Quebec, Canada.

References

1. Alberti KG, Zimmet PZ: Definition, diagnosis, and classification of diabetes mellitus and its complications, part 1: diagnosis and classification of diabetes mellitus: provisional report of a WHO consultation. *Diabet Med* 1998;15:539-553.

2. Puavilai G, Chanprasertyotin S, Sriphrapradaeng A: Diagnostic criteria for diabetes mellitus and other categories of glucose intolerance: 1997 criteria by the Expert Committee on the Diagnosis and Classification of Diabetes Mellitus (ADA), 1998 WHO consultation criteria, and 1985 WHO criteria. World Health Organization. *Diabetes Res Clin Pract* 1999;44:21-26.

3. Third Report of the National Cholesterol Education Program (NCEP) Expert Panel on Detection, Evaluation, and Treatment of High Blood Cholesterol in Adults (Adult Treatment Panel III). US Department of Health and Human Services. National Institutes of Health. National Heart, Lung, and Blood Institute. NIH Publication No. 02-5215. September 2002.

4. Report of the National Cholesterol Education Program Expert Panel on Detection, Evaluation, and Treatment of High Blood Cholesterol in Adults: the Expert Panel. *Arch Intern Med* 1988;148:36-69.

5. Castelli WP, Garrison RJ, Wilson PW, et al: Incidence of coronary heart disease and lipoprotein cholesterol levels. The Framingham Study. *JAMA* 1986;256:2835-2858.

6. Hulley S, Ashman P, Kuller L, et al: HDL-cholesterol levels in the Multiple Risk Factor Intervention Trial (MRFIT) by the MRFIT Research Group 1,2. *Lipids* 1979;14:119-123.

7.   Stamler J, Wentworth D, Neaton JD: Is relationship between serum cholesterol and risk of premature death from coronary heart disease continuous and graded? Findings in 356,222 primary screenees of the Multiple Risk Factor Intervention Trial (MRFIT). *JAMA* 1986;256:2823-2828.

8.   Horenstein RB, Smith DE, Mosca L: Cholesterol predicts stroke mortality in the Women's Pooling Project. *Stroke* 2002; 33:1863-1868.

9.   The Lipid Research Clinics Coronary Primary Prevention Trial results. I. Reduction in incidence of coronary heart disease. *JAMA* 1984;251:351-364.

10.   The Lipid Research Clinics Coronary Primary Prevention Trial results. II. The relationship of reduction in incidence of coronary heart disease to cholesterol lowering. *JAMA* 1984;251:365-374.

11.   Manolio TA, Pearson TA, Wenger NK, et al: Cholesterol and heart disease in older persons and women. Review of an NHLBI workshop. *Ann Epidemiol* 1992;2:161-176.

12.   Silberberg JS, Henry DA: The benefits of reducing cholesterol levels: the need to distinguish primary from secondary prevention. 1. A meta-analysis of cholesterol-lowering trials. *Med J Aust* 1991;155:665-666, 669-670.

13.   Holme I: Cholesterol reduction in single and multifactor randomized trials: relationship to CHD incidence and total mortality as found by meta analysis of twenty-two trials. *Blood Press* 1992;4:29-34.

14.   Rossouw JE, Lewis B, Rifkind BM: The value of lowering cholesterol after myocardial infarction. *N Engl J Med* 1990;323: 1112-1119.

15.   The Expert Committee of the Diagnosis and Classification of Diabetes Mellitus: Follow-up report on the diagnosis of diabetes mellitus. *Diabetes Care* 2003;26:3160-3167.

16.   National Institutes of Health: Clinical guidelines on the identification, evaluation, and treatment of overweight and obesity trials in adults—the evidence report. Bethesda, MD, National Heart, Lung, and Blood Institute. NIH Publication no. 98-4083. 1998. 228 pages.

17.   Balkau B, Charles MA: Comment on the provisional report from the WHO consultation. European Group for the Study of Insulin Resistance (EGIR). *Diabet Med* 1999;16:442-433.

18. Chandalia M, Abate N, Garg A, et al: Relationship between generalized and upper body obesity to insulin resistance in Asian Indian men. *J Clin Endocrinol Metab* 1999;84:2329-2335.

19. Dogadin SA, Nozdratchev KG: Prevalence of type 2 diabetes and other metabolic syndrome components in northern indigenous population of Siberia. Available at: http://www.diabetolognytt.nu/abstracts2000/393.pdf.

20. Lee J, Heng D, Chia KS, et al: Risk factors and incident coronary heart disease in Chinese, Malay and Asian Indian males: the Singapore Cardiovascular Cohort Study. *Int J Epidemiol* 2001;30: 983-988.

21. Hughes K, Aw TC, Kuperan P, et al: Central obesity, insulin resistance, syndrome X, lipoprotein(a), and cardiovascular risk in Indians, Malays, and Chinese in Singapore. *J Epidemiol Community Health* 1997;51:394-399.

22. Ward AM, Fall CH, Stein CE, et al: Cortisol and the metabolic syndrome in South Asians. *Clin Endocrinol (Oxf)* 2003;58: 500-505.

23. Vasan RS, Larson MG, Leip EP, et al: Impact of high-normal blood pressure on the risk of cardiovascular disease. *New Engl J Med* 2001;345:1291-1297.

24. Panza, JA: High-normal blood pressure–more 'high' than 'normal.' *New Engl J Med* 2001;345:1337-1340.

25. The Seventh Report of The Joint National Committee on Prevention, Detection, Evaluation, and Treatment of High Blood Pressure. US Department of Health and Human Services, National Institutes of Health, National Heart, Lung, and Blood Institute, National High Blood Pressure Education Program. NIH Publication No. 03-5233, May 2003.

26. American Diabetes Association: Clinical practice recommendations 1998: screening for type 2 diabetes. *Diabetes Care* 1998;21 (suppl 1):S1-S98.

27. World Health Organization: Definition, diagnosis and classification of diabetes mellitus and its complications: Report of a WHO Consultation. Part 1. Diagnosis and classification of diabetes mellitus. Geneva, World Health Organization, 1999. Available at: http://whqlibdoc.who.int/hq/1999/WHO_NCD_NCS_99.2.pdf. Accessed February 26, 2004.

28. Reaven GM: Banting lecture 1988. Role of insulin resistance in human disease. *Diabetes* 1988;37:1595-1607.

29.   Reaven GM, Lerner RL, Stern MP, et al: Role of insulin in endogenous hypertriglyceridemia. *J Clin Invest* 1967;46:1756-1767.

30.   Laws A, Reaven GM: Evidence for an independent relationship between insulin resistance and fasting plasma HDL-cholesterol, triglyceride and insulin concentrations. *J Intern Med* 1992;231:25-30.

31.   Reaven GM, Chen YD, Jeppesen J, et al: Insulin resistance and hyperinsulinemia in individuals with small, dense low density lipoprotein particles. *J Clin Invest* 1993;92:141-146.

32.   Ferrannini E, Haffner SM, Mitchell BD, et al: Hyperinsulinemia: the key feature of a cardiovascular and metabolic syndrome. *Diabetologia* 1991;34:416-422.

33.   Abbasi F, Brown BW Jr, Lamendola C, et al: Relationship between obesity, insulin resistance, and coronary heart disease risk. *J Am Coll Cardiol* 2002;40:937-943.

34.   Bogardus C, Lillioja S, Mott DM, et al: Relationship between degree of obesity and in vivo insulin action in man. *Am J Physiol* 1985;248(3 Pt 1):E286-E291.

35.   Matthews DR, Hosker JP, Rudenski AS, et al: Homeostasis model assessment: insulin resistance and β-cell function from fasting plasma glucose and insulin concentrations in man. *Diabetologia* 1985;28:412-419.

36.   Hanley AJ, Williams K, Stern MP, et al: Homeostasis model assessment of insulin resistance in relation to the incidence of cardiovascular disease: The San Antonio Heart Study Diabetes Care, July 1, 2002;25:1177-1184.

37.   Einhorn D, Reaven GM, Cobin RH, et al: American College of Endocrinology position statement on the insulin resistance syndrome. *Endocr Pract* 2003;9:237-252.

38.   Ford ES, Giles WH, Dietz WH: Prevalence of the metabolic syndrome among US adults: findings from the third National Health and Nutrition Examination Survey. *JAMA* 2002;287:356-359.

39.   Meigs JB, Wilson PW, Nathan DM, et al: Prevalence and characteristics of the metabolic syndrome in the San Antonio Heart and Framingham Offspring Studies. *Diabetes* 2003;52:2160-2167.

40.   Grundy SM, Brewer HB Jr, Cleeman JI, et al: Definition of metabolic syndrome: Report of the National Heart, Lung, and Blood Institute/American Heart Association conference on scientific issues related to definition. *Circulation* 2004;109:433-438.

41. Richard JL, Sultan A, Daures JP, et al: Diagnosis of diabetes mellitus and intermediate glucose abnormalities in obese patients based on ADA (1997) and WHO (1985) criteria. *Diabet Med* 2002;19:292-299.

42. Lemieux I, Pascot A, Couillard C, et al: Hypertriglyceridemic waist: A marker of the atherogenic metabolic triad (hyperinsulinemia; hyperapolipoprotein B; small, dense LDL) in men? *Circulation* 2000;102:179-184.

43. St-Pierre J, Lemieux I, Vohl MC, et al: Contribution of abdominal obesity and hypertriglyceridemia to impaired fasting glucose and coronary artery disease. *Am J Cardiol* 2002;90:15-18.

44. Lemieux I, Almeras N, Mauriege P, et al: Prevalence of 'hypertriglyceridemic waist' in men who participated in the Quebec Health Survey: association with atherogenic and diabetogenic metabolic risk factors. *Can J Cardiol* 2002;18:725-732.

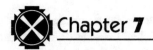 **Chapter 7**

Lifestyle Modification: First-line Approach to the Metabolic Syndrome

The promotion of lifestyle changes should be the first-line approach to management or prevention of the metabolic syndrome. Specific guidelines have been developed for treatment of major risk factors, and these may require drug therapies. However, adoption of lifestyle changes, particularly before atherosclerotic cardiovascular disease (ASCVD) and diabetes have developed, can go a long way toward the prevention of these complications.

Although unalterable genetic factors affect each person, the right combination and intensity of lifestyle improvements can have a significant impact on outcome. For this reason, and the fact that an estimated one fourth of all Americans are at risk for or already have significant manifestations of the metabolic syndrome, a public health approach promises the greatest good for the greatest number.

Previous chapters have dealt with definition and early detection of the components of the metabolic syndrome in clinical and investigative settings. This chapter examines the multiple nonpharmaceutical avenues for primary and secondary prevention. In all cases, prevention and treatment overlap because of the cumulative nature of the disease processes. Pharmaceutical interventions are the subject of several subsequent chapters. But lifestyle changes are the foundation on which other approaches are built.

Public Health Approach

The goals of the public health approach to preventing ASCVD and diabetes are fourfold: foster healthy eating habits, encourage weight control, tout the benefits of physical activity, and strongly advocate for the avoidance of smoking and for smoking cessation. Much of the reduction in ASCVD in the United States in the past 50 years can be ascribed to the success of the public health approach. Smoking among men has declined by almost half. The intake of animal fats and cholesterol, chief components of an unhealthy diet, have declined substantially. Both changes have contributed to reducing ASCVD. Unfortunately, the rise in obesity and sedentary habits of Americans have had the opposite effect on the prevalence of the metabolic syndrome and type 2 diabetes. While the dietary and smoking messages need constant reinforcement, the problems of obesity and lack of exercise constitute a public health crisis. Consequently, all of the approaches to public health education need to be mobilized: government, media, academia, educational institutions, industry, and health organizations.

Unfortunately, neither the full magnitude of the risks of the metabolic syndrome nor the extent of the lifestyle changes required are appreciated.

Increasing awareness is only a first step, but an important one. Advertisers know that it takes multiple repetitions of a message for it to sink in, annoying as it is sometimes. Health messages are no exception. Public service announcements in the media, advertisements for products that address the issue (even if the products themselves are ineffective), news reports of new discoveries or treatment approaches, and advice and encouragement from physicians all have a place in increasing public awareness.

Combined Lifestyle Therapies

Because the metabolic syndrome is a clustering of factors variously woven into each person's profile, therapeutic interventions must be multifactorial, cumulative, and individualized to suit each patient's unique makeup. The result will be the product of incremental changes. Fortunately, each increment is measurable and will provide patients with reinforcement and encouragement to maintain the change and to make other changes. A key principle for physicians to remember when urging patients to adopt healthier lifestyles is that the patient is the senior partner in all negotiations and must be complicit in them for progress to be made. Therefore, the first step is to agree on goals and the need to achieve them.

The priority given to each change will be determined individually with the help of risk data and the patient's profile.

Behavioral Changes

An effective nonpharmacologic, behavioral approach to reducing the impact of the metabolic syndrome on health combines four targets: smoking cessation, weight loss, increased physical activity, and dietary modification. The ultimate goal is an entirely new lifestyle, something that is unlikely to be achieved by anything other than a progressive approach, one step at a time. Fortunately, each step carries its own rewards, so that the motivation that is all-important in pursuing the goal can be reinforced at each interval.

A behavioral modification program is based on the urgency of modifying each behavior, the patient's motivation to do so, the support and follow-through available, and the patient's overall health status. Patients should be encouraged to design an overall program at the outset, complete with a reasonable timetable for each phase—a master plan, if you will. Setting a goal, having it in writing, and maintaining a commitment offer real benefits. Such a plan identifies the problem and its magnitude, outlines a plan of action, specifies the requirements for fulfilling each step, and provides a checklist of accomplishments (Table 7-1).

Table 7-1: Behavioral Changes for a Better Lifestyle

Goal	Requirements	Time to completion
Weight loss	10% reduction in body weight in 1 year	1.5 lb/wk
Quit smoking	Freedom	30 days
Diet optimization	ATP III guidelines	60 days
Exercise	Regular routine at least 30 min 5 x/wk at 80% maximum pulse rate	Check calendar diary for compliance every month
Clear kitchen of junk food	None left	Tomorrow

How to Achieve Behavioral Changes

Physicians should emphasize the lifestyle changes set forth by Adult Treatment Panel III (ATP III) as the first and most important intervention for patients with or at risk for the metabolic syndrome. Specific strategies to identify risk factors as early as possible will contribute strongly to individual awareness of the immediacy of the threat. Because risk varies substantially by population group, it is also reasonable to identify specific risks and their magnitude in identifiable subpopulations, tailoring screening recommendations and early interventions to each group.

The Role of Physicians

Periodic health checkups, which are already recommended for both sexes and all ages, include a history of important symptoms and predispositions, vital signs, a physical examination, and minimal laboratory work, perhaps a urinalysis and hematocrit. Various cost-benefit analyses have been done for many elements of a routine physical, most recommending Pap smears and mammography for at-risk women, and prostate-specific antigen (PSA) test for older men.[1,2] For healthy adults, a serum lipoprotein panel should be obtained at least once every 5 years. Blood pressure levels should be measured every 2 years, or more frequently for elevations, as outlined in JNC 7. If a person has two or more major risk factors, Framingham Heart Study risk scoring should be performed.

The physician's participation is required for behavior modification success. The patient will look to the physician for guidance, but equally important, the physician's attitude is crucial. Unfortunately, many physicians have a negative attitude about the prospects for behavior modification. They tend to be overly influenced by those patients who fail to make meaningful changes. But millions of people have successfully modified their life habits to improve their health, including patients who have stopped smoking, have started and maintained an exercise program, or have successfully lost weight. Also, the decline in average cholesterol level in the general population attests to a widespread change in diet. For these reasons, a positive and encouraging outlook is essential. Physician participation in behavior modification requires a few minutes with the patient to take a proper history and make the appropriate referrals. Many physicians are so concerned with the reason for a patient's visit that they do not take the time to look to the patient's future health. Unless this is achieved, behavior modification may never start.

Nurses, Physician Assistants, and Nurse Practitioners

Nurses and other health-team professionals usually spend more time in patient contact than physicians do. They frequently interpret physicians' treatment recommendations, particularly when patients are discharged from the hospital. They maintain contact with patients, have the chance to advocate lifestyle and compliance recommendations, and can estimate risk using Framingham risk scores when given the necessary laboratory values.

Dietitians/Nutritionists

Nutrition professionals are greatly underused as resources who can help patients with, or at risk for, the metabolic syndrome. The important role they play in hospitals and on nutritional research teams should be extended more often to individual patient counseling. Patient referral to intensive and comprehensive dietary services can provide invaluable assistance to menu planners. Ethnic food preferences require a high diversity of expertise to counsel heterogeneous populations.

If dietary goals for lifestyle changes are not met after a few physician visits, counseling by a nutritional professional is strongly encouraged. Considering the cost, safety, and efficacy of professional nutritional counseling compared with medical/surgical interventions, few arguments can be raised against such a recommendation.

Dietitians can go beyond menus to effect behavioral change. They should emphasize improved eating habits (such as setting realistic goals, planning meals systematically, selecting healthy foods by reading labels, avoiding eating binges, avoiding snacks, and reducing portions).

Weight Reduction

Goal of Therapy

A defined goal of weight reduction should be set for overweight/obese patients with the metabolic syndrome.[3,4] Clinical trials indicate that a reasonable goal is to achieve a reduction in body weight of 10% in 6 months to 1 year. For example, a person who weighs 220 lb should strive to reduce his or her weight to 200 lb in the first year. Then, a decision can be made on whether further weight loss is required. The decision will be based primarily on the response in metabolic risk factors. Studies have shown that much of the benefit of reducing these risk factors can be achieved with the reduction of 10% of body weight, which is realistic and practical for many patients.

Long-term weight loss and successful maintenance at a more desirable weight require self-discipline. A number of habits are associated with overeating. Table 7-2 lists suggestions for acquiring improved eating habits.

Overeating is frequently used to relieve emotional stress. Others eat when they are lonely or sad. Keeping a diary of eating habits can be helpful. Included in the diary should be foods eaten, when, and how much. Physical activity can be recorded in the same diary. Sharing information with others may reveal overlooked patterns. Once identified, such stimuli can be resisted. Self-talk can serve to restructure a person's attitudes toward eating (ie, telling oneself, 'Oh, that tastes good but is bad for me. I'd rather get into that bathing suit next summer.').

Low-Calorie Diets

A reduction in caloric intake is required for weight reduction. There have been two persistent questions about such diets: (1) how low should the calorie count be? and (2) what should be the composition of a low-calorie diet in obese persons?

To achieve a weight loss of about 25 lb in 6 months, it is necessary to reduce caloric intake by about 500 calories per day. This change will result in a weight reduction of approximately 1 pound per week.[3,4] Many people, however, desire to 'jump-start' the weight reduction process. They prefer to reduce calories by about 1,000 calories per day. To get this jump-start, women should reduce calories to a maximum of 1,200 per day, and men should not exceed 1,800 calories per day. The downside of extreme reduction in calories is that the focus is placed more on caloric deficit than on behavior modification. Only through behavior modification will it be possible to achieve long-term weight reduction. Therefore, more emphasis should be placed on behavior modification than on calorie counting for long-term weight reduction.

Table 7-2: Behavioral Changes That Will Facilitate Weight Reduction

- Snacking—Eat in only one place, at the dining table.

- Nibbling—Eliminate nibbles from the house.

- Junk food—Throw it out and do not buy more.

- Too much—Control the portions that you eat. Spend longer tasting each bite.

- Dining out—No buffets. Choose soups and salads (easy on the creamy salad dressings) and appetizers or side dishes rather than entrees with all the trimmings.

- In the grocery store—Buy only what is on your list. Do not shop when you are hungry.

- At parties—Ask for the vegetable hors d'oeuvres (without the creamy dressing).

- At cocktail parties—Sip your alcohol slowly. You get just one.

Tips for Resisting Temptation

- Change your typical driving route to avoid the fast food and donut places, or other venues that typically tempt you on the road.

Motivation

- Give away all clothing that is too big for you. Repeat every 6 months.

- Share your efforts with others. Group encouragement is powerful.

- Reward yourself (not with food) for each 5 lb lost.

Many 'weight reduction' diets are advocated and promoted. Most of these are extreme diets that emphasize rapid weight reduction. They are not the types of diet that people can follow for the rest of their lives. Some of these diets are very low in fat. Others promote reduction of carbohydrates. A diet that is reduced in fat and carbohydrates so that the relative amounts left in the diet are balanced is preferred. Thus, even if a major caloric deficit is used to jump-start the process, a combined reduction of fats and carbohydrates will make it easier to achieve a long-term, healthy diet.

There are several drawbacks to extreme reductions in calories, even when used for short periods. Experience shows that most people who experience rapid weight loss without behavior modification will return to their previous weights. This often causes a sense of failure and depression. Many obese persons will undergo repeated cycles of weight loss and weight gain. Some health experts believe that weight cycling is detrimental to long-term health. Finally, the likelihood of developing cholesterol gallstones is increased in patients who follow a severely reduced caloric diet.

Increased Physical Activity as a Weight Reduction Adjunct

Including increased exercise in a weight-reduction regimen offers several advantages.[3,4] As examined later in the chapter, exercise helps to mitigate the metabolic risk factors in addition to its effect on weight reduction. Furthermore, it promotes energy expenditure and can contribute 2% to 3% of body weight reduction.

Weight Reduction Drugs

Two types of weight reduction drugs are available for clinical use.[3] One is an appetite suppressant, the other reduces fat absorption. The only approved drug to inhibit appetite is sibutramine (Meridia®), a serotonin and noradrenaline reuptake inhibitor. Sibutramine generally is well tolerated, though in some patients it causes dry mouth, anorexia, and insomnia. The major concern is in patients with hypertension; it can raise blood pressure, which is worrisome in patients at risk for ASCVD. In short-term trials of weight-reduction diets, sibutramine can produce an additional 5% reduction in body weight in more than half the subjects. An unresolved question is whether it can be used for a lifetime. Clinical trials have been too short to answer this question. Therefore, long-term trials are required to determine its place in the treatment of obesity.

Orlistat (Xenical®) inhibits the absorption of fat, operating in the gut to inhibit intestinal lipase. Unhydrolyzed dietary fat cannot be absorbed and consequently is excreted. When given at the recommended dose (120 mg 3 times daily), this drug reduces fat absorption by approximately 30%. Short-term clinical trials show that orlistat will reduce body weight about 4% beyond what can be achieved by low-calorie diets. Fat malabsorption (steatorrhea) is an unacceptable side effect in some patients. Again, whether efficacy and tolerability persist over many years has not been tested.

Bariatric Surgery

Gastrointestinal (GI) surgery to produce weight loss has gained popularity among some obese patients in the United States. Many patients choose bariatric surgery because they may feel socially rejected and psychologically depressed, or as part of a regimen to help cope with severe medical problems, such as diabetes. Rapid weight reduction in obese persons greatly increases the risk for gallstone formation. Careful, thorough evaluation of patients for bariatric surgery is required. Selection of patients for surgery should follow existing guidelines.[5]

A variety of procedures have been used, including gastric banding, vertical banded gastroplasty, Roux-en-Y gastric bypass, biliopancreatic diversion, duodenal switch, and laparoscopic adjustable gastric banding.

Generally, weight reductions achieved by bariatric surgery are much greater and longer lasting than those obtained by dietary modification. However, side effects of surgery are greater than those occurring with dietary change. Among the side effects reported are intestinal leak, pulmonary embolus, GI hemorrhage, stenosis of the GI tract, and wound infections. Some patients undergoing bariatric surgery go into pulmonary failure, and this complication appears to be more common in smokers. Although there appears to be a place for bariatric surgery in the management of severe obesity and its complications, it should be performed only where there is a clear need to deal with severe medical or psychological complications.

Diet Composition During and After Weight Reduction

Millions of overweight people commonly believe that if they could just find the 'right' diet they would lose weight. This view is bolstered and promoted by commercial interests. Through the years, many diet books have been advertised and sold. Most of the recommended diets are extreme, restrictive, and favor the use of just a few foods or types of foods. Two currently popular are low-fat diets and low-carbohydrate diets. Others identify a small range of 'acceptable' foods. Unfortunately, most people who adopt extreme diets regain the weight they lose. The claim that extreme diets are useful to jump-start successful weight reduction has not been proved.

As a rule, the composition of a weight reduction diet should resemble as closely as possible the diet that the patient will eventually follow daily. Behavior modification should begin immediately, and the patient's acquired eating habits should be used in the long run as well as the short run.

In choosing a short-term and long-term eating pattern, a few principles should be followed.[2,3] Because obesity typically is accompanied by eating too much fat and carbohydrates, both need to be reduced, especially animal fats, because they raise the serum cholesterol level. Vegetable oils or soft margarines are preferable. There are many sources of excessive carbohydrates in the diet of obese persons. These should be identified and reduced or avoided. The diet should be liberal in fruits and vegetables. The fat percentage in the diet depends on personal preference; it can range from 25% to 35% of calories.

Two dietary patterns have been identified in epidemiologic studies as being associated with low rates of ASCVD.[6] These are the Mediterranean diet and the Asian diet. The Mediterranean diet is characterized by low intake of animal fat, liberal consumption of olive oil, and large amounts of vegetables and fruits, pasta, and fish. It is low in carbohydrate and high in vegetable oil. The traditional Asian diet is low in both animal and vegetable fats but much higher in carbohydrates. Rice is the primary source of carbohydrate.

The low rates of ASCVD observed in Mediterranean and Asian countries may have been due partly to heavy physical activity and a lack of obesity. Both diets appear to be well tolerated under these conditions. However, the Asian diet could raise concern because in persons with the metabolic syndrome, it can accentuate metabolic risk factors. The Mediterranean diet may be preferable in the presence of the metabolic syndrome, although obesity and physical inactivity can override its potential benefits.

Whether patients are following a weight-reduction diet or a weight-maintenance diet, a few principles should be observed for diet composition. These are summarized, with the rationale for the recommendations.

Saturated fats. In cross-population studies, higher intakes of saturated fats are accompanied by increased risk for ASCVD. The reason appears to be that saturated fats raise the serum low-density lipoprotein (LDL)-cholesterol level, one of the chief culprits for cardiovascular disease.[7]

A 1% change in saturated fatty acid intake in either direction will produce a corresponding 1% to 2% change in serum cholesterol level, making saturated fats a major determinant of LDL cholesterol levels.[7,8] Although it is not possible to remove all saturated fats from the diet, intake should be reduced to less than 10% of total calories for the general public and to less than 7% for persons at risk for ASCVD. The major sources of saturated fats in the diet are dairy products (butter, whole milk, cheese, ice cream, cream); animal fats (lard, tallow, marbled meat, hamburger, ground meat); processed meats (sausage, salami, frankfurters, bologna); tropical oils (palm oil, coconut oil, and palm kernel oil); baked products and mixed dishes containing dairy fat and tropical oils.

Trans fats. These fats are unsaturated but have a double bond in the trans configuration. They are produced by hydrogenation of polyunsaturated oils, a process that raises their melting points and turns liquids into solids at room temperature. The trans fats raise LDL-cholesterol levels similarly to saturated fatty acids.[7,8] The typical American diet contains 2% to 4% of total calories as trans fatty acids. Common sources of trans fatty acids are shortenings and hard margarines; bakery goods made with shortenings (cakes and pies); foods prepared with shortenings (eg, French fries); and milk fat.

Dietary cholesterol. The third LDL-raising nutrient of the diet is cholesterol. The American diet normally contains 300 to 500 mg/d of cholesterol. A cholesterol-lowering diet for the general public should be reduced to <300 mg/d, but persons at risk for ASCVD should reduce intake to <200 mg/d. The major sources of dietary cholesterol are egg yolks (240 mg/egg); dietary fats (especially milk fat products); and meat.

In a typical American diet, intake of dietary cholesterol is about equally divided among these three sources.

Unsaturated fats. The harmless unsaturated fats are of three types: *cis*-monounsaturated, N-6 polyunsaturated, and N-3 polyunsaturated. The typical American diet contains 25% to 30% of total calories as unsaturated fats. Unsaturated fats do not raise the LDL-cholesterol level and thus are preferred over saturated fats. Animal fats are rich in monounsaturated fats, so when saturated animal fats are reduced, monounsaturated fats are, too. In the Mediterranean region, which has a high intake of monounsaturated fat (olive oil), the prevalence of ASCVD is low.[6]

The other major source of unsaturated fats is plant oils. Oils that are particularly rich in monounsaturated fatty acids include olive oil, canola oil, and high-oleic safflower oil.

N-6 polyunsaturated fats are derived exclusively from plant sources. Clinical trials have shown that enriching the diet with N-6 polyunsaturated fats at the expense of saturated fats will produce lower serum cholesterol levels and fewer major coronary events.[9] Usual sources are corn oil, safflower oil, and soybean oil.

N-3 polyunsaturated fatty acids can come from either fish oils or plant oils. The N-3 polyunsaturates in fish oil consist of eicosapentaenoic acid (EPA) (20:5) and docosahexaenoic acid (DHA) (22:6). Those from plant oils consist mostly of linolenic acid. The diet normally contains about 1% of total calories as N-3 fatty acids. These fatty acids may have special biologic properties that may protect against ASCVD or its complications and are now under study.[9] Some investigators advocate using 1 g/d N-3 fatty acids in patients with established ASCVD to prevent fatal arrhythmias.[10]

Carbohydrates. There are two main types of carbohydrates: sugars (monosaccharides and disaccharides) and polysaccharides (starches and fiber). The typical diet contains 45% to 55% of calories as carbohydrates. Although it was previously thought that high intake of carbohydrates is without adverse effects, recent evidence suggests that overconsumption of carbohydrates contributes to obesity.[9] Moreover, high-carbohydrate diets can raise triglyceride levels, reduce high-density lipoprotein (HDL) cholesterol levels, and enhance postprandial responses to glucose and insulin.[6] High intake can thus be detrimental in people with the metabolic syndrome.[11]

To prevent these responses and to promote weight control, patients must pay attention to the sources of carbohydrates. Some investigators have identified particular carbohydrate-rich foods that may give an exaggerated postprandial glucose response. These foods are called high-glycemic index foods. These include bread, processed cereals, cookies and crackers, potatoes, and rice. Even so, when these foods are consumed in mixed-food meals, some of their hyperglycemic action may be attenuated.

Common sources of excess sugar in the diet are soft drinks, fruit juices, cookies, cakes, pies, honey, and syrup. Simple sugars are also present in skim milk and fruits, although potentially useful nutrients are contained in these foods as well. Common sources of excess polysaccharides are rice, bread, potatoes, pasta, and grains. Many nutritionists prefer whole grains as a carbohydrate source because they contain fiber as well as digestible starch. High intake of fiber is widely advocated because it can reduce the glycemic response and may lower serum cholesterol levels.

Good sources of high-fiber foods are fruits, vegetables, whole grains, dried beans, and oat bran. Psyllium bulk laxatives are also a good source of fiber. Viscous fiber (eg, fiber in oats, pectin, guar, psyllium, and beans), but not insoluble fiber (eg, bran and cellulose fiber), can modestly reduce LDL cholesterol.[10]

Protein. Many animal and plant products are good sources of protein, such as lean meat and skim milk. Sources of animal protein that are lower in saturated fat and cholesterol include fat-free and low-fat dairy products, egg whites, fish, skinless poultry, and lean meats. Soy and other vegetable proteins can supply adequate nutrition without the accompanying animal fats. Despite claims to the contrary, the amount and quality of protein have little effect on plasma LDL-C levels. High intake of soy protein has been reported to lower LDL-C levels, but the effect is small.

Plant stanols/sterols. Esters of plant stanols and sterols at dosages of 2 g/d can lower LDL-C levels by 6% to 15% when incorporated into margarines and similar fat-containing products.[12-18] Stanol esters are preferable to sterol esters because they are absorbed to a lesser extent. Plant stanol esters can be recommended as part of an LDL-lowering diet.

Antioxidants. Studies of the antioxidants ascorbic acid (vitamin C), α-tocopherol (vitamin E), β-carotene, ubiquinone (coenzyme Q10), bioflavonoids, and selenium in cardiovascular disease have produced mixed results, even though oxidation of LDL appears to be an important step in the development of atherosclerosis. Population studies support the contention that diets rich in fruits, vegetables, and other foods high in antioxidants are associated with decreased risk of CHD. Controlled clinical trials, however, have been equivocal.[19-22] On the basis of results in laboratory animals and small clinical studies, antioxidants appear to offer potential for long-term reduction of risk for ASCVD.

Alcohol. Observational, case-control, cohort, and ecologic studies indicate a J-curve relationship between alcohol consumption and CHD risk. These studies indicate that 1/2 to 1 oz of ethanol a day in any form is associated with lower risk for CHD.[23-25] Whether alcohol prevents CHD remains uncertain. Because higher doses are convincingly associated with substantial risk of multiple disease states, health claims for alcohol, if any, must be disseminated with great care to a nation of 20 million to 30 million people suffering from alcohol abuse.

Sodium, potassium, and calcium. Lowering salt intake to 2,400 mg or 1,800 mg/d can lower blood pressure and may reduce risk for hypertension.[26-30] The diet that contains many of the benefits listed above—high in fruits and vegetables, low-fat dairy products, whole grains, poultry, fish, and nuts and low in fats, red meat, and sweets—is also rich in potassium, calcium, and magnesium. Such a diet lowers blood pressure even without a change in salt intake,[30] and more so if the two interventions are combined.[31]

Neutraceuticals. There is great public interest in the neutraceuticals, as well as in complementary and alternative medicine. Unfortunately, accumulating convincing evidence in a field as complex as the metabolic syndrome requires enormous expenditures of time, effort, and money. Disinterested parties, such as the National Institutes of Health, are just beginning to explore the gathering of the necessary data to investigate the claimed benefits of neutraceuticals.

Physical Activity

Physical inactivity is a major risk factor for CHD.[32] Every component of the metabolic syndrome benefits from exercise. Lipid levels improve; HDL is elevated; VLDL is lowered, and often, LDL is also lowered. Blood pressure falls; insulin resistance declines; glycogen synthesis and insulin-stimulated glucose uptake are enhanced;[33] insulin-independent glucose transport increases (mediated in part by AMP-activated protein kinase[34]); and cardiovascular capacity increases along with coronary blood flow. At the same time, morphologic changes and increased capillary supply in muscle tissue shift fuel requirements to fat, reducing glycolytic flux and acid-base fluctuations. Taken collectively, these adaptations result in enhanced performance capacity and lower demands on insulin/glucose metabolism.[35,36]

Most people can devise their own exercise programs with minimal guidelines from health professionals. Perhaps the most important advice concerns duration and intensity. The minimum effort to improve cardiovascular fitness appears to be in the range of 30 minutes of exercise 4 to 5 times a

Table 7-3: Caloric Expenditure by Activity

Activity	Cal/h	Activity	Cal/h
Sleep	80	Biking	210
Sitting	100	Walking	210
Driving	120	Gardening	220
Fishing	130	Golf	250
Standing	140	Swimming	300
Housework	180	Jogging	585

week at 70% of age-adjusted maximum pulse rate. Clinicians can advise 30 minutes of brisk walking or raking leaves, 15 minutes of running, or 45 minutes of playing volleyball on most, if not all, days of the week. Maximum heart rate can be calculated by this formula:

Women	**Men**
209 minus age x 0.7	214 minus age x 0.8

Wrist pulse monitors are available commercially. A few patients, such as those with autonomic neuropathy from diabetes, cannot increase their pulse rates normally and require expert exercise counseling to establish a safe and effective routine. Patients with cardiac disease or other limitations on physical activity will benefit from professional exercise advice to devise the safest and most effective programs.

It is often claimed that aerobic exercise, more than other forms of exercise, improves cardiorespiratory fitness and endurance. Aerobic exercise maintains an established oxygen deficit throughout and can theoretically be continued indefinitely. Anaerobic exercise is a degree of exertion that continues to increase the oxygen deficit, such as sprinting while holding one's breath. It does not last long. For

Table 7-4: Tobacco-related Health Problems

- A smoker is 2 to 6 times more likely to have a heart attack or stroke; the greater the tobacco use, the higher the risk.

- Smoking increases risk for cancers of the mouth, larynx, pharynx, esophagus, lung, stomach, pancreas, kidney, breast, bladder, and cervix.

- Respiratory diseases linked to tobacco use include chronic obstructive pulmonary disease, emphysema, chronic bronchitis, bronchial asthma, and hay fever.

- Surgeons found poorer healing among smokers; some will not perform spinal fusion on smokers because their spines do not fuse. Some plastic surgeons refuse to perform cosmetic surgery on smokers because of poor results.

- Female smokers have a unique set of risks:
  - Smoking greatly elevates the risk of heart attack and stroke in women taking birth-control pills.
  - Women who smoke during pregnancy are more likely to have a miscarriage, stillbirth, or baby with a low birth weight.
  - There is a direct relationship between smoking during pregnancy and sudden infant death syndrome (SIDS).
  - Smoking in pregnancy may be responsible for as many as 10% of all infant deaths in the United States.
  - Other increased risks for female smokers include high blood pressure and circulation problems, and an increased risk of developing osteoporosis and its attendant risk for bone fractures.

- Men experience more erectile dysfunction and impotence.
- Additional associated conditions for *both* sexes include:
  - Gastroesophageal reflux disease, peptic ulcer disease, and ulcerative colitis
  - Renal diseases
  - Age-related macular degeneration, glaucoma, and cataract
  - Gingivitis and periodontal diseases
  - Gray hair and baldness
  - Premature wrinkles
  - Infertility in men and women
  - Weakened immune system
  - Sore eyes, sore throat
  - Headaches
  - Overall decreased life expectancy

Table 7-5: Methods That Sometimes Help Patients to Stop Smoking

- Nicotine replacement—pills, patches, and lozenges in a variety of formulations and dosing schedules aim to replace the addictive chemical in tobacco, breaking the multiple social and habit patterns associated with smoking before weaning the smoker from the drug itself. Nicotine replacement is an effective addition to smoking cessation programs and has been credited with a significant success rate.

- Tapering—as with any addiction, stringing out withdrawal allows the body to readapt to its drug-free state gradually, with fewer symptoms. A rigid schedule is required, and intense personal monitoring greatly enhances the success rate. One recommended schedule is to ration a declining daily number of cigarettes each morning and lock up the rest.

cardiovascular conditioning, aerobic exercise is recommended, but muscular strengthening by weight lifting or progressive resistance training has additional benefits.

One rule about exercise applies universally: 'If you don't like it, you won't do it.' Tips to increase activity include parking farther away from your destination and walking, using stairs instead of elevators, using hand-operated tools instead of power tools (eg, lawnmowers), and finding an active hobby such as swimming or tennis. The caloric expenditure for a variety of activities is listed in Table 7-3.

- Bupropion (Zyban®) has been approved by the Food and Drug Administration for smoking cessation. How Zyban® works is largely unknown, but it claims a 1-year success rate of 30% in a comprehensive cessation program, and 35% when nicotine replacement is added.[39]

- Pearls:

  - Cost—a patient's motivation can be increased by calculating the patient's cost of the smoking habit.

  - Halfway measure—one of the best ideas to initiate a cessation program is to encourage the smoker to throw away half of each cigarette. Many of the toxins in tobacco are removed by the filter as the smoke passes through it, so the second half of the cigarette is far more pathogenic than the first half. Ask the patient to draw a line around the middle of each cigarette and discard it after smoking to the line.

Smoking Cessation

There is little disagreement on the overriding importance of smoking cessation in preventing cardiovascular disease. Tobacco is the leading preventable cause of death and disease in the United States. The literature is full of examples of the benefits of smoking cessation.[37,38] Cigarette smoke contains more than 4,000 chemicals, including ammonia, arsenic, carbon monoxide, DDT, formaldehyde, and nitric acid. At least three of these compounds are known carcinogens. To date, tobacco has been identified as the cause of, or a major contributor to, 29 diseases, including ASCVD. Table 7-4 is a comprehensive list of tobacco-related health problems.

Nicotine is addictive. Withdrawal symptoms may last for weeks. Addicts who have successfully abandoned cocaine, heroin, amphetamines, psychedelics, and sedatives still have difficulty giving up smoking. On the brighter side, many smokers have been able to quit, using one or more of the many available methods.

The principal ingredient behind all successful smoking programs is motivation. Repetition is the keystone to effective motivation. There is no better place to start than showing a patient the list of smoking-related diseases (Table 7-4). Fear motivates—perhaps it is the most effective motivator. A list of methods that have been shown to be effective in smoking cessation appears in Table 7-5.

To convince patients that smoking cessation is necessary, the clinician must overcome their objections. Perhaps the greatest obstacle, particularly in overweight patients, is the patient's fear of weight gain. Eighty percent of quitters will gain an average of 4.5 to 7 lb, but 13% of women and 10% of men will gain more than 28 lb.[40-42] Women are particularly intimidated by this problem.[43] The best and perhaps only response to this objection is simply that smoking is a greater risk to health in many more ways than excess body weight.[44] A third of the weight gain associated with smoking cessation appears to be because of a decrease in the resting metabolic rate of 100 cal/d.[41,45,46] The remaining two thirds comes from increased caloric intake,[46,47] the result of improved ability to taste food. This weight gain is more resistant to dietary counseling than other forms of overweight.[48,49] Various drugs, including nicotine phenylpropanolamine and bupropion, delay postcessation weight gain, but their effect does not persist after discontinuation.

Long-term weight loss is possible. A key decision to make is whether to institute weight loss and smoking cessation simultaneously or sequentially.

References

1.   Battista RN: Practice guidelines for preventive care: the Canadian experience. Canadian Task Force on the Periodic Health Examination. *Br J Gen Pract* 1993;43:301-304.

2.   The periodic health examination: age-specific charts. US Preventive Services Task Force. *Am Fam Physician* 1990;41:189-204.

3.   National Institutes of Health: Clinical guidelines on the identification, evaluation, and treatment of overweight and obesity in adults—the evidence report. Bethesda, MD, National Heart, Lung, and Blood Institute. NIH Publication no. 98-4083. 1998. 228 pages.

4.   Grundy SM, Hansen B, Smith SC Jr, et al: Clinical management of metabolic syndrome: report of the American Heart Association/National Heart, Lung, and Blood Institute/American Diabetes Association conference on scientific issues related to management. *Circulation* 2004;109:551-556.

5.   NIH conference. Gastrointestinal surgery for severe obesity. Consensus Development Conference Panel. *Ann Intern Med* 1991;115:956-961.

6.   Grundy SM: The optimal ratio of fat-to-carbohydrate in the diet. *Annu Rev Nutr* 1999;19:325-341.

7.   Grundy SM, Denke MA: Dietary influences on serum lipids and lipoproteins. *J Lipid Res* 1990;31:1149-1172.

8.   Mensink RP, Katan MB: Effects of dietary fatty acids on serum lipids and lipoproteins: A meta-analysis of 27 trials. *Arterioscler Thromb* 1992;12:911-919.

9.   US Department of Agriculture, US Department of Health and Human Services: Nutrition and your health: dietary guidelines for Americans. 5th ed. Washington, DC, US Department of Agriculture. Home and Garden Bulletin no. 232. 2000. 44 pages.

10.   Grundy SM: N-3 fatty acids: priority for post-myocardial infarction clinical trials. *Circulation* 2003;107:1834-1836.

11.   Grundy SM, Abate N, Chandalia M: Diet composition and the metabolic syndrome: what is the optimal fat intake? *Am J Med* 2002;113(suppl 9B):25S-29S.

12.   Hallikainen MA, Uusitupa MI: Effects of 2 low-fat stanol ester-containing margarines on serum cholesterol concentrations as part of a low-fat diet in hypercholesterolemic subjects. *Am J Clin Nutr* 1999;69:403-410.

13. Gylling H, Miettinen TA: Cholesterol reduction by different plant stanol mixtures and with variable fat intake. *Metabolism* 1999;48:575-580.

14. Gylling H, Radhakrishnan R, Miettinen TA: Reduction of serum cholesterol in postmenopausal women with previous myocardial infarction and cholesterol malabsorption induced by dietary sitostanol ester margarine: women and dietary sitostanol. *Circulation* 1997;96:4226-4231.

15. Hendriks HF, Weststrate JA, van Vliet T, et al: Spreads enriched with three different levels of vegetable oil sterols and the degree of cholesterol lowering in normocholesterolaemic and mildly hypercholesterolaemic subjects. *Eur J Clin Nutr* 1999;53:319-327.

16. Miettinen TA, Puska P, Gylling H, et al: Reduction of serum cholesterol with sitostanol-ester margarine in a mildly hypercholesterolemic population. *N Engl J Med* 1995;333:1308-1312.

17. Vanhanen HT, Blomqvist S, Ehnholm C, et al: Serum cholesterol, cholesterol precursors, and plant sterols in hypercholesterolemic subjects with different apoE phenotypes during dietary sitostanol ester treatment. *J Lipid Res* 1993;34:1535-1544.

18. Vuorio AF, Gylling H, Turtola H, et al: Stanol ester margarine alone and with simvastatin lowers serum cholesterol in families with familial hypercholesterolemia caused by the FH-North Karelia mutation. *Arterio Thromb Vasc Biol* 2000;20:500-506.

19. The effect of vitamin E and beta carotene on the incidence of lung cancer and other cancers in male smokers. The Alpha-Tocopherol, Beta Carotene Cancer Prevention Study Group. *N Engl J Med* 1994;330:1029-1035.

20. Hennekens CH, Buring JE, Manson JE, et al: Lack of effect of long-term supplementation with beta carotene on the incidence of malignant neoplasms and cardiovascular disease. *N Engl J Med* 1996;334:1145-1149.

21. Omenn GS, Goodman GE, Thornquist MD, et al: Effects of a combination of beta carotene and vitamin A on lung cancer and cardiovascular disease. *N Engl J Med* 1996;334:1150-1155.

22. Stephens NG, Parsons A, Schofield PM, et al: Randomised controlled trial of vitamin E in patients with coronary disease: Cambridge Heart Antioxidant Study (CHAOS). *Lancet* 1996;347:781-786.

23. Criqui MH: Alcohol and coronary heart disease: consistent relationship and public health implications. *Clinica Chimica Acta* 1996;246:51-57.

24. Criqui MH: Alcohol and hypertension: new insights from population studies. *Eur Heart J* 1987;(suppl B):19-26.

25. Dufour MC: If you drink alcoholic beverages do so in moderation: what does this mean? *J Nutr* 2001;131(2S-1):552S-561S.

26. The sixth report of the Joint National Committee on prevention, detection, evaluation, and treatment of high blood pressure. *Arch Intern Med* 1997;157:2413-2446.

27. Chobanian AV, Bakris GL, Black HR, et al: Seventh report of the Joint National Committee on Prevention, Detection, Evaluation, and Treatment of High Blood Pressure. *Hypertension* 2003;42:1206-1252.

28. National Research Council: Diet and health: implications for reducing chronic disease risk. Washington, DC, National Academy Press, 1989, pp 171-120.

29. Chobanian AV, Hill M: National Heart, Lung, and Blood Institute Workshop on Sodium and Blood Pressure: a critical review of current scientific evidence. *Hypertension* 2000;35:858-863.

30. Appel LJ, Moore TJ, Obarzanek E, et al: A clinical trial of the effects of dietary patterns on blood pressure. DASH Collaborative Research Group. *N Engl J Med* 1997;336:1117-1124.

31. Sacks FM, Svetkey LP, Vollmer WM, et al: Effects on blood pressure of reduced dietary sodium and the Dietary Approaches to Stop Hypertension (DASH) diet. DASH-Sodium Collaborative Research Group. *N Engl J Med* 2001;344:3-10.

32. Fletcher GF, Balady G, Blair SN, et al: Statements on exercise: benefits and recommendations for physical activity programs for all Americans: a statement for health professionals by the Committee on Exercise and Cardiac Rehabilitation of the Council on Clinical Cardiology, American Heart Association. *Circulation* 1996;94:857-862.

33. Sakamoto K, Goodyear LJ: Invited review: intracellular signaling in contracting skeletal muscle. *J Appl Physiol* 2002;93:369-383.

34. Zierath JR: Invited review: Exercise training-induced changes in insulin signaling in skeletal muscle. *J Appl Physiol* 2002;93:773-781.

35.   Hawley JA: Adaptations of skeletal muscle to prolonged, intense endurance training. *Clin Exp Pharmacol Physiol* 2002;29:218-222.

36.   US Department of Health and Human Services: Physical activity and health: a Report of the Surgeon General. Atlanta, Georgia: US Department of Health and Human Services, Centers for Disease Control and Prevention, National Center for Chronic Disease Prevention and Health Promotion, 1996, 278 pages.

37.   Jorenby DE, Leischow SJ, Nides MA, et al: A controlled trial of sustained-release bupropion, a nicotine patch, or both for smoking cessation. *N Engl J Med* 1999;340:685-691.

38.   Gerace TA, Hollis J, Ockene JK, et al: Smoking cessation and change in diastolic blood pressure, body weight, and plasma lipids. MRFIT Research Group. *Prev Med* 1991;20:602-620.

39.   Klesges RC, Meyers AW, Klesges LM, et al: Smoking, body weight, and their effects on smoking behavior: a comprehensive review of the literature. *Psychol Bull* 1989;106:204-230.

40.   Williamson DI, Madans J, Anda RI, et al: Smoking cessation and severity of weight gain in a national cohort. *N Engl J Med* 1991;34:739-745.

41.   Pirie PL, Murray DM, Luepker RV: Gender differences in cigarette smoking and quitting in a cohort of young adults. *Am J Public Health* 1991;81:324-327.

42.   Pomerleau GS, Kurth CL: Willingness of female smokers to tolerate postcessation weight gain. *J Subst Abuse* 1996;8:371-378.

43.   Perkins KA, Epstein LH, Marks BL, et al: The effect of nicotine on energy expenditure during light physical activity. *N Engl J Med* 1989;320:898-903.

44.   Stamford BA, Matter S, Fell RD, et al: Effects of smoking cessation on weight gain, metabolic rate, caloric consumption, and blood lipids. *Am J Clin Nutr* 1986;43:486-494.

45.   Spring B, Wurtman J, Gleason R, et al: Weight gain and withdrawal symptoms after smoking cessation: a preventive intervention using d-fenfluramine. *Health Psychol* 1991;10:216-223.

46.   Gilbert RM, Pope MA: Early effects of quitting smoking. *Psychopharmacology (Berl)* 1982;78:121-127.

47.   Hurt RD, Sachs DP, Clover ED, et al: A comparison of sustained-release bupropion and placebo for smoking cessation. *N Engl J Med* 1997;337:1195-1202.

48.   Hall SM, Tunstall CD, Vila KL, et al: Weight gain prevention and smoking cessation: cautionary findings. *Am J Public Health* 1992;82:799-803.

49.   Gross J, Stitzer ML, Maldonado J: Nicotine replacement: effects of postcessation weight gain. *J Consult Clin Psychol* 1989;57: 87-92.

Chapter 8

Atherogenic Dyslipidemia

Atherogenic dyslipidemia is a consistent component of the metabolic syndrome in many populations. It consists of the following lipid abnormalities in the serum:

- elevations of apolipoprotein B (apo B)
- elevations of triglyceride-rich lipoproteins (TGRLP)
- elevations of small low-density lipoprotein (LDL) particles
- low high-density lipoprotein (HDL) cholesterol.

All of these abnormalities enhance the risk for atherosclerotic cardiovascular disease (ASCVD). Thus, management of atherogenic dyslipidemia is critical for the appropriate management of the metabolic syndrome. First-line treatment of atherogenic dyslipidemia is therapeutic lifestyle changes (TLC); however, if abnormalities persist after lifestyle therapies, drug therapy may be required.

Goals of Lipid-lowering Therapy

The goals of therapy for each of the components of atherogenic dyslipidemia have been identified in the National Cholesterol Education Program Adult Treatment Panel III (NCEP ATP III) report and the recent update of the ATP III report.[1,2] Each can be reviewed briefly as it pertains to persons with the metabolic syndrome.

Elevations of Apolipoprotein B-containing Lipoproteins

There are three potential targets of therapy among the apo B-containing lipoproteins: LDL cholesterol, very low-density lipoprotein (VLDL) + LDL (non-HDL) cholesterol, and total apo B. ATP III defines goals of therapy according to a patient's risk status for coronary heart disease (CHD).[1] In those with isolated elevations of LDL, serum LDL cholesterol is a sufficient target of treatment. However, in those with other components of atherogenic dyslipidemia, as is typical of the metabolic syndrome, the other components should be included in therapy. According to ATP III, even in patients with the metabolic syndrome, LDL cholesterol remains the primary target of therapy. However, when atherogenic dyslipidemia is identified, usually by elevation of triglyceride (TG) levels, VLDL+LDL cholesterol becomes a secondary target. The total apo B can be used as an alternative to VLDL+LDL cholesterol. Table 8-1 shows suggested goals of treatment for different categories of risk.

For high-risk patients, the LDL-cholesterol goal is <100 mg/dL (Table 8-1). According to ATP III, conditions of high CHD risk are established CHD, including history of myocardial infarction, unstable angina, stable angina, coronary artery procedures, or clinical evidence of myocardial ischemia; noncoronary forms of ASCVD (eg, peripheral arterial disease, abdominal aortic aneurysm, clinical carotid artery disease); diabetes; and multiple (2+) risk factors with 10-year risk for major coronary events (myocardial infarction + coronary death) >20%. In a patient with the metabolic syndrome, VLDL+LDL cholesterol becomes an important secondary goal of therapy. The goal for VLDL+LDL cholesterol is <130 mg/dL.[1] If apo B is used as an alternate secondary target, the goal is <90 mg/dL.[3] VLDL+LDL cholesterol is highly correlated with total apo B and represents an adequate target of therapy when accurate measures of total apo B are not available. Few studies support apo B as a preferred target over VLDL+LDL cholesterol.

Based on recent clinical trials, the ATP III update[2] introduced the concept of an optional LDL-cholesterol goal

Table 8-1: Treatment Goals for LDL Cholesterol, VLDL+LDL Cholesterol, and Total Apo B

Risk Status	Primary Target: LDL Cholesterol Therapeutic Goal (mg/dL)
High risk Very high risk	<100 mg/dL Optional <70 mg/dL
Moderately high risk (2+ risk factors* and 10-year risk 10% to 20%)	<130 mg/dL (optional: <100 mg/dL)
Moderate risk (2+ risk factors and 10-year risk <10%)	<130 mg/dL
Lower risk (0-1 risk factor)	<160 mg/dL

* Risk factors include cigarette smoking, hypertension (blood pressure >140/90 mm Hg or on antihypertensive medication), low HDL cholesterol (<40 mg/dL), family history of premature CHD (CHD in first-degree male relative <55 years; CHD in first-degree female relative <65 years), and age (men >45 years; women >55 years).

for patients at very high risk for CHD. Four recent studies suggest that reducing LDL cholesterol to well below 100 mg/dL may further reduce risk in very high risk patients.[4-7] The general dictum 'the lower, the better' seems to hold for LDL cholesterol in very high risk patients, but physicians must use clinical judgment when applying it. A di-

Secondary Target: VLDL+LDL Cholesterol** Therapeutic Goal (mg/dL)	Secondary Target: Total Apo B*** Therapeutic Goal (mg/dL)
<130 mg/dL Optional <100 mg/dL	<90 mg/dL
<160 mg/dL (optional: <130 mg/dL)	<110 mg/dL
<160 mg/dL	<110 mg/dL
<190 mg/dL	<130 mg/dL

** VLDL+LDL cholesterol (non-HDL-cholesterol) becomes a secondary goal of therapy when serum TG levels range from 200 to 500 mg/dL. It is calculated as total cholesterol minus HDL.

*** Apo B is an alternative secondary goal of therapy when serum TG levels range from 200 to 500 mg/dL.

agnosis of very high risk should be considered in patients with established cardiovascular disease (CVD) plus (a) multiple major risk factors (especially diabetes), (b) severe and poorly controlled risk factors (especially continued cigarette smoking), or (c) multiple risk factors of the metabolic syndrome (especially elevated TG >200 mg/dL plus non-HDL-C >130 mg/dL with low HDL-C <40 mg/dL) or recent acute coronary syndromes. Presumably, the VLDL+LDL cholesterol goal would be correspondingly lower if the lower goal for LDL cholesterol is set. To date, there are no data on obtaining very low apo B goals.

For patients with 2+ major risk factors in the moderately high risk or moderate-risk categories, the therapeutic goal for LDL cholesterol is <130 mg/dL.[1] Corresponding goals for VLDL+LDL cholesterol and total apo B are <160 mg/dL and <110 mg/dL, respectively. The ATP III update introduced an optional LDL-cholesterol goal of <100 mg/dL for patients with moderately high CHD risk (2+ risk factors and 10-year risk 10% to 20%). This option is to be exercised though clinical judgment, and it will presumably be reserved for those who are approaching the high-risk category. When 0 to 1 risk factor is present, the LDL-cholesterol goal is <160 mg/dL, while the goals for VLDL+LDL and total apo B are <190 mg/dL and <130 mg/dL, respectively. When persons with the metabolic syndrome have 0 to 1 major risk factor, an effort should be made to achieve these goals of treatment using TLC without drugs.

Elevated Triglyceride Levels

According to ATP III, when TG is elevated, VLDL+LDL cholesterol levels (or total apo B) become secondary targets of therapy. In ATP III, the TG cut point for adding these secondary treatment targets is 200 mg/dL. However, it is reasonable to introduce these measures as secondary targets when persons have TG levels >150 mg/dL plus the metabolic syndrome. Triglycerides become a direct target of lipid-lowering therapy only when levels exceed 500 mg/dL. When TG levels are very high, the risk for acute pancreatitis increases. Triglyceride-lowering therapy must then be introduced. The goal is to reduce TG levels to <500 mg/dL, a level that will not cause pancreatitis. When TG is in the range of 150 to 499 mg/dL, VLDL remnants represent a risk factor. However, elevations of remnant lipoproteins are identified in the VLDL+LDL cholesterol fraction. Therefore, therapies for TG in this range are better directed against VLDL+LDL cholesterol (or total apo B) rather than against elevated TG.

Small LDL Particles

Although small LDL particles probably introduce added risk to the metabolic syndrome, they generally do not represent unique targets of therapy, according to ATP III. Elevations of small LDL particles contribute to higher levels of VLDL+LDL cholesterol and total apo B. Thus, they are included among all of the apo B-containing lipoproteins that are the secondary targets of treatment. In short, LDL cholesterol is the primary target of therapy, and VLDL+LDL cholesterol (including total apo B and small LDL particles) is a secondary target. There are two ways that small LDL particles can be changed to reduce CHD risk: reducing their number or converting them to larger LDL. Therapies reducing TG levels usually lead to a conversion of smaller to larger LDL.[8]

Low HDL Levels

ATP III identifies a low HDL-cholesterol level as a tertiary target of treatment, after LDL cholesterol and non-HDL cholesterol. Although low HDL-cholesterol levels are highly predictive of risk for CVD, there is little clinical trial evidence that therapies directed toward raising HDL cholesterol reduce risk. For this reason, ATP III does not specify a particular goal for HDL. Although increasing HDL levels may protect against atherosclerosis, the evidence is scant to make specific recommendations. However, the pharmaceutical industry is heavily engaged in efforts to develop new and more effective HDL-raising drugs. If such drugs can be shown to reduce risk, they undoubtedly would find a place in the treatment of atherogenic dyslipidemia.

Therapeutic Lifestyle Changes for Atherogenic Dyslipidemia

First-line therapy of atherogenic dyslipidemia is management of underlying risk factors with TLC, as examined in Chapter 7. However, special consideration can be given to lifestyle changes as they pertain to management of atherogenic dyslipidemia.

Weight Reduction and Increased Physical Activity

A 10% reduction in body weight usually produces a significant decrease in TG levels.[9,10] Often, TG can be normalized if body weight is reduced to the desirable range. However, in persons with a significant genetic component of atherogenic dyslipidemia, weight loss may not adequately normalize TG levels. In particular, weight reduction often will not normalize HDL-cholesterol concentrations. But even if drug therapy is required for management of atherogenic dyslipidemia, efficacy will be enhanced by concomitant weight reduction. Likewise, increased physical activity will promote weight reduction and reduce insulin resistance. Both weight reduction and increased physical activity will improve the lipid profile and enhance efficacy if drugs are required.

Low-carbohydrate Diets

There is growing interest in the use of low-carbohydrate diets for improvement of the lipid profile and for weight reduction.[11] Extremely low-carbohydrate diets for weight reduction are a problem, however, because of difficulty in long-term adherence. Moderate reductions in carbohydrates may be useful for achieving long-term weight reduction. Additionally, moderate reductions tend to lower TG levels and raise HDL-cholesterol levels. In such diets, the percentage of fat may rise (eg, 35% of total calories).[1] A fat intake equal to 35% of total calories is acceptable, provided that animal fats and trans-fats are reduced. Most dietary fatty acid should come from monounsaturated and polyunsaturated fatty acids.

Drug Therapies for Atherogenic Dyslipidemia

Drugs That Primarily Reduce Apo B-containing Lipoproteins and VLDL+LDL Cholesterol

The hydroxymethyl glutaryl coenzyme A (HMG CoA) reductase inhibitors (statins) are highly effective drugs for

Table 8-2: LDL-Cholesterol Average Reduction With Standard Doses of Available Statins

Drug	Dose (mg/d)	LDL reduction (%)
Atorvastatin (Lipitor®)	10	39
Fluvastatin (Lescol®)	40-80	25-31
Lovastatin (Mevacor®)	40	31
Nicotinic acid/lovastatin (Advicor®)	1,000/40	36
Pravastatin (Pravachol®)	40	34
Rosuvastatin (Crestor®)	5-10	39-45
Simvastatin (Zocor®)	20-40	35-41

reducing apo B-containing lipoproteins. They primarily lower LDL levels but also lower atherogenic remnant lipoproteins. Numerous clinical trials document the efficacy of statins for reducing risk in higher-risk patients.[1] No single trial has exclusively tested patients with the metabolic syndrome, but subgroup analysis of the major statin trials strongly suggests that these drugs reduce risk for CVD in these patients.[12] Statins have proved generally safe in clinical practice. Six statins are available in clinical practice; these are listed in Table 8-2 along with standard doses and average LDL-cholesterol reductions.

One other statin, cerivastatin, was removed from the market because it proved to have a side effect/efficacy ratio that was too high to sustain its use in clinical practice.

Mechanisms of statin action

Statins lower apo B-containing lipoproteins by increasing hepatic expression of LDL receptors. Normally, statins act almost exclusively in the liver. They reduce the synthesis of cholesterol by inhibiting hepatic HMG CoA reductase.[13,14] This action lowers the cholesterol content of liver cells, which in turn increases the synthesis of LDL receptors. LDL receptors interact with circulating lipoproteins containing apo B. They mediate the removal of these lipoproteins (LDL and VLDL remnants) from the circulation. Statins given in high doses may also reduce the secretion of lipoproteins by the liver.

The dose-response relationship between statin dose and LDL lowering is not proportional. Generally, for every doubling of the dose of statins, LDL cholesterol concentrations fall by another 6%. Thus, tripling the dose lowers LDL-cholesterol levels by about 12%, and quadrupling the dose, by 18%. However, the dose of statin required to produce various reductions of LDL varies. A standard dose of statin is one that produces a 30% to 40% reduction of LDL cholesterol.

Some investigators believe that statins have a beneficial effect on CVD risk beyond lowering apo B-containing lipoproteins (pleiotropic effects).[15] Examples of suggested pleiotropic effects include anti-inflammation, antithrombosis, reduced cellular proliferation, and improved vascular reactivity. Several of these effects have been reported in the literature. However, whether they are secondary to lowering of atherogenic lipoproteins or to other actions has not been determined. Moreover, comparing the risk reductions obtained in statin trials to those obtained with other cholesterol-lowering modalities suggests that benefits are always proportional to LDL lowering.[1] This observation makes any lipoprotein-independent action unlikely to be substantial.

Major clinical trials with statins

Major clinical trials with statin therapy have reported a reduction in ASCVD.[1] Disease reductions include acute coronary syndromes (unstable angina, myocardial infarction, and coronary death), coronary procedures, various other coronary outcomes, and stroke. Statin therapy reduces new-onset and recurrent CVD events. Because of these trials, statins have emerged as first-line cholesterol-lowering therapy. Clinical trials typically are separated into primary and high-risk (secondary) prevention trials. Two studies, the Heart Protection Study (HPS)[4] and the Prospective Study of Pravastatin in the Elderly at Risk (PROSPER),[16] included patients at high risk with and without ASCVD. These trials will be listed with the high-risk prevention trials.

Three primary prevention trials of statin therapy are the West of Scotland Coronary Prevention Study (WOSCOPS),[17] the Air Force/Texas Coronary Atherosclerosis Prevention Study (AFCAPS/TexCAPS),[18] and the Anglo-Scandinavian Cardiac Outcomes Trial—Lipid Lowering Arm (ASCOT-LLA) (Table 8-3).[19] In all three trials, statin treatment significantly reduced relative risk (RR) for major coronary events. In WOSCOPS, a strong trend toward a decrease in total mortality was observed. In AFCAPS/TexCAPS and ASCOT, the number of deaths was too small to draw any conclusions about effects of statin therapy on total mortality. Nonetheless, no increase in noncardiovascular mortality was observed. In fact, even nonfatal adverse effects were rare.

Similar reductions in RR for ASCVD events were obtained in high-risk patients in secondary prevention trials. However, there was a greater benefit for higher-risk patients because of their higher absolute risk. The results of the trials from high-risk patients are summarized in Table 8-4. New trials published since publication of ATP III are HPS[4] and PROSPER.[16]

In these trials, statin therapy was efficacious for all types of patients. Similar reductions in RR were observed for men vs women, older vs younger patients, smokers vs non-smokers, hypertensives vs normotensives, and patients with diabetes vs those without. Several subgroup analyses of clinical trials have documented in considerable detail the benefits of statins in these subgroups. Of particu-

Table 8-3: Major Primary Prevention Trials With Statins (Modified From ATP III Report)

Study	Patients	Duration
WOSCOPS	6,595	4.9 yr
AFCAPS/ TexCAPS	6,605	5 yr
ASCOT-LLA	10,305	3.3 yr

Study	Major Coronary Events	Revascularization
WOSCOPS	-31%*	-37%*
AFCAPS/ TexCAPS	-37%*	-33%*
ASCOT-LLA	-29%*	

*Changes significant at *P* <0.05 or lower.

WOSCOPS = West of Scotland Coronary Prevention Study, AFCAPS/TexCAPS = Air Force/Texas Coronary Atherosclerosis Prevention Study, ASCOT-LLA = Anglo-Scandinavian Cardiac Outcomes Trial—Lipid-Lowering Arm

lar interest is the substantial RR in patients with diabetes. This benefit has been reported for 4S,[20] CARE,[21] and HPS.[4]

There is controversy, however, about whether patients at all baseline levels of LDL obtain the same reduction in RR with statin therapy.[23] One problem with this analysis is that baseline levels of LDL cholesterol are not stable, and assigning patients to the correct category of baseline

Statin Drug (dose/d)	Baseline LDL-C (mg/dL)	LDL-C Change	Coronary Mortality	Total Mortality
pravastatin 40 mg	192	-26%*	-33%*	-22%*
lovastatin 20/40 mg	150	-25%*	NS	NS
atorvastatin 10 mg	132	-32%*		NS

NS = not significant

LDL may not be accurate. Nonetheless, the recent HPS strongly suggested that even those with very low LDL levels at entry into the trial received benefit from further LDL lowering.[4]

Side effects of statin therapy

Statins, like almost all other drugs, are not entirely free of side effects. Occasionally, patients will have gastro-

Table 8-4: Major Secondary Prevention Trials With Statins: Morbidity and Mortality Results (Modified From ATP III Report)

Study	Patients	Duration
4S[20]	4,444	5.4 yr
CARE[21]	4,159	5 yr
LIPID[22]	9,014	5 yr
HPS	20,536	5 yr
PROSPER	5,804	3.2 yr

Study	Major Coronary Events	Revascularization
4S[20]	-35%*	-37%*
CARE[21]	-25%*	-27%*
LIPID[22]	-29%*	-24%*
HPS	-27%	-24%
PROSPER	-19%*	NA

*Statistically significant changes at $P<0.05$ or lower.
4S = Scandinavian Simvastatin Survival Study,
CARE = Cholesterol and Recurrent Events,
LIPID = Long-term Intervention with Pravastatin in
Ischaemic Disease, HPS = Heart Protection Study,

Drug (dose/d)	Baseline LDL-C (mg/dL)	LDL-C Change	Coronary Mortality	Total Mortality	Stroke
simvastatin 10/40 mg	188	-35%*	-42%*	30%*	-27%*
pravastatin 40 mg	139	-27%*	-24%*	-9%*	-31%*
pravastatin 40 mg	150	-25%*	-24%*	-23%*	-19%*
simvastatin 40 mg	131	-29%	-18%	-17%	-25%
pravastatin 40 mg	146	-34%	NS	NS	NS

PROSPER = Prospective Study of Pravastatin in the Elderly at Risk
NS = not significant

Table 8-5: Classification of Statin-induced Myopathy

Myopathy category	Symptoms
Mild	Myalgia
	With or without myalgia
Moderate	Myalgias
Severe	Muscle pain and weakness

intestinal (GI) complaints or will manifest skin or allergic reactions. Insomnia has been reported but has been difficult to verify in specific studies. The same is true for nonspecific weakness and myalgia. Some patients respond to statin therapy, particularly at higher doses, with elevations of hepatic transaminases. The major concern, although rare, is myopathy.[24]

The clinical significance of elevated serum transaminases is uncertain. The major concern, of course, is hepatotoxicity. That statins cause liver injury by predisposing people to cirrhosis or chronic liver disease is doubtful; there is no documentation. Some authorities believe that modest rises in transaminases are a physiologic response to the drug and do not indicate true hepatotoxicity. Routine monitoring of liver function tests for patients on statin therapy seems to be unnecessary.

However, statins can definitely cause myopathy. The author's classification of statin-induced myopathy is shown in Table 8-5.

Complaints of myalgia with statin therapy are relatively common. Although many patients and physicians believe in statin-induced myalgias, clinical trials have not verified their existence. The frequencies of such complaints in placebo and statin-treated groups are similar. In clinical practice, physicians should take a patient's complaints

Creatine Kinase

No elevation

Elevation <3x normal

Elevations 3x-10x normal

Elevations >10x normal

---

seriously and work through them with the goal of maintaining statin therapy. Frequently, the complaint can be shown to relate to another condition (eg, arthritis, tendonitis). Switching to another statin sometimes eliminates the complaint, as does lowering the dose. Some physicians try supplements (coenzyme Q or L-carnitine), with some apparent success. Whether these adjuncts are placebos or actually reduce muscle symptoms is open to question. Other patterns of statin use, such as starting at low doses and working up as tolerated or using alternate-day therapy, may be successful.

The development of moderate but persistent elevations of creatine kinase (CK) requires attention. If these elevations can be shown to be caused by statin treatment, the drug may need to be discontinued. Nonetheless, it must be remembered that other causes elevate CK (eg, other muscle disease, mild forms of trauma). African Americans often normally exhibit what would be considered moderate elevations in whites. Finally, the procedures listed above for myalgias can be tried in patients with moderate CK elevations with the aim of maintaining effective therapy.

Severe myopathy is the most feared side effect of statin therapy. It is characterized by muscle pain and weakness, CK elevations >10 times normal, and brown urine (myoglobinuria). The latter can cause acute renal failure, which may result in death. An unacceptably high frequency of severe myopathy and renal failure led to the removal of cerivastatin from the market. Certain risk factors predict the development of severe myopathy (Table 8-6).[24]

For patients with the metabolic syndrome, the combination of statin + gemfibrozil (Lopid®) significantly increases risk for myopathy. This risk is much lower when a statin is combined with fenofibrate (TriCor®, Lofibra™). However, when this combination is used, avoid high doses of statins. Generally, statin therapy should be avoided or doses kept low in patients who have risk factors for statin-induced myopathy.

Clinical indications of statin therapy in patients with the metabolic syndrome

Any person who is eligible for therapy to achieve treatment goals for LDL cholesterol, VLDL+LDL cholesterol, or total apo B is a candidate for statin therapy (Table 8-1). Among the apo B-lowering drugs, statins are usually preferred because they are highly efficacious and well tolerated. They are especially useful for high-risk patients (Table 8-1). Beyond this, however, because of growing evidence of risk reduction and safety, statins are being used increasingly in persons at intermediate risk and even those at lower risk who have severe hypercholesterolemia. A high proportion of subjects at high and intermediate risk will manifest the metabolic syndrome. Strong evidence supports statin use in higher-risk patients with the metabolic syndrome, including those with type 2 diabetes.

Add-on LDL-lowering Drugs to Statin Therapy

Although statins represent primary therapy for reducing LDL, VLDL+LDL, and apo B, standard doses often fail to achieve the goals of therapy outlined in Table 8-1. One approach to attaining the therapeutic goal is to increase the dose of the statin. For every doubling of the statin dose, the LDL-cholesterol level will be reduced by

Table 8-6: Risk Factors for Severe Myopathy

- Older people who are frail or have a small body frame, especially older women

- Presence of multisystem disease (especially debilitated status)

- Chronic renal insufficiency (including diabetic renal disease)

- Chronic liver disease

- Hypothyroidism

- Coadministration of multiple medications, particularly gemfibrozil, cyclosporine, azole antifungals (itraconazole and ketoconazole), macrolide antibiotics (erythromycin and clarithromycin), HIV protease inhibitors, the antidepressant nefazodone, and verapamil.

- Severe illnesses and perioperative periods. Statins should usually be withheld when patients are admitted to the hospital for acute illnesses or for major surgery.

- Alcohol abuse

- Heavy exercise

- Daily consumption of large quantities of grapefruit juice (eg >1 quart per day)

approximately 6%. In uncomplicated individuals, high doses of statins are usually well tolerated, and the goals of therapy are often achieved. However, in persons who carry risk factors for severe myopathy, the standard dose of statin usually should not be exceeded. This includes the concomitant use of fibrates such as fenofibrate. In such cases, the goals of therapy may better be attained by using LDL-lowering drugs in combination. Among the latter, the cholesterol-absorption blockers and the bile acid absorption blockers are most frequently used.

Cholesterol-absorption blockers

One category of cholesterol-absorption blockers is the plant stanols and sterols. These are naturally occurring sterols found in plants and incorporated into two margarines (Benecol® and Take Control®). In a dose of about 2 g/d, they will reduce LDL-cholesterol levels by 10% to 15%[25,26] and enhance the LDL reduction achieved by dietary means. They further reduce LDL-cholesterol levels in individuals taking statins.

Another cholesterol-absorption blocker is ezetimibe (Zetia®),[27,28] which typically lowers LDL-cholesterol levels by 15% to 22%. The drug was recently released on the market and appears to be safe, with no serious side effects reported. When ezetimibe is combined with standard doses of statins, an additional 15% to 22% reduction in LDL-cholesterol levels can be obtained. This equates to a quadrupling of the statin dose. Ezetimibe is an attractive agent for use in combination with statins in patients with the metabolic syndrome, in whom high doses of statins may not be acceptable.[27,28]

Bile acid absorption blockers

Bile acid absorption blockers were among the first available LDL-lowering drugs.[1] They bind to bile acids in the intestine and thus prevent reabsorption. Blocking return of bile acids to the liver releases feedback inhibition, promoting conversion of cholesterol to bile acids in the liver. Thus, more cholesterol is converted into bile acids, and hepatic cholesterol concentrations fall. This stimulates the synthesis of LDL receptors, which in turn lowers serum LDL levels. Depending on the dose of bile acid absorption blocker, the LDL level can be reduced by 15% to 30%. When moderate doses of these agents are added to statin therapy, the LDL level usually falls by an additional 15% to 20%, equivalent to quadrupling the dose of statin. The efficacy of bile acid absorption blockers in reducing the risk for CHD was demonstrated in the Lipid Research Clinics Coronary Prevention Trial.[29] In this trial, a 1% reduction in LDL-cholesterol levels reduced risk for major coronary events by at least 1%, similar to statin therapy.

Three bile acid absorption blockers are available for therapy: cholestyramine (Prevalite®), colestipol (Colestid®), and colesevelam (Welchol®). Moderate doses of the first two are 8 and 10 g/d, respectively. Colesevelam is a new bile acid absorption blocker that is effective for LDL reduction in lower doses than similar agents.[30] The usual dose of colesevelam is 3.75 g/d. It is the author's impression that bile acid absorption blockers in combination with statins are underused in patients who have difficulty in achieving the goals of therapy with statins alone.

The major reason for avoiding the use of bile acid absorption blockers is concern about toleration of side effects. These drugs act exclusively in the GI tract, where they can produce upper GI distress or constipation, both of which usually abate with continued use. Constipation can usually be prevented by taking a psyllium-based bulking agent. Early research suggested that bile acid absorption blockers also could block the absorption of other drugs (eg, digoxin, warfarin, thyroxine, thiazide diuretics, β-blockers). Therefore, these agents should not be administered simultaneously with the blocker, but at a different time. Bile acid absorption blockers can raise TG levels, so they should be avoided in patients with severe hypertriglyceridemia. They can, however, be used in patients with mild elevations of TG, such as those with type 2 diabetes.[31]

Drugs That Primarily Reduce Triglyceride-rich Lipoproteins and Raise HDL Cholesterol

In persons with the metabolic syndrome, LDL cholesterol remains the primary target of therapy. The first priority of therapy is to achieve the goals for LDL, VLDL+LDL, and apo B (Table 8-1). For most persons who require drug therapy, LDL-lowering drug(s) will be needed. Even so, many persons with the metabolic syndrome will still have elevated TG and/or reduced HDL-cholesterol levels after the primary goals are achieved. In these persons, the physician can consider starting a drug that mainly reduces TGRLP or raises HDL cholesterol. These drugs are nicotinic acid and fibrates. Usually, one of these drugs will be add-on therapy to statin treatment.

Fibric acid derivatives (fibrates)

Although fibrates were once considered useful only for severe hypertriglyceridemia, their use has been increasing, for several reasons. There is growing acceptance of their efficacy because of controlled clinical trials; they are attractive for use in persons with atherogenic dyslipidemia and the metabolic syndrome; they are well tolerated and generally safe; and much has been learned about their mechanisms of action.

The three fibrates available in the United States are clofibrate (Atromid-S®), gemfibrozil, and fenofibrate.

Clofibrate is rarely used anymore. Other fibrates with similar actions are available, however. Although gemfibrozil has been the most widely used fibrate in the United States, use of fenofibrate is growing. Fenofibrate seemingly has the advantage of safety when used in combination with a statin, which makes it an attractive choice for patients with the metabolic syndrome.

Effects of fibrates on lipid and lipoprotein metabolism. Fibrates have multiple effects on lipid and lipoprotein metabolism. All of these effects appear to be secondary to fibrates' action as agonists of the nuclear receptor, peroxisome proliferator-activated receptor α (PPAR α).[32] One of the major tissue locations of PPAR α is the liver, which is where fibrates have their major lipid effects. The following actions have been reported for lipid metabolism in the liver with fibrate administration: peroxisomal proliferation in rodents promoting fatty acid oxidation[33]; increased mitochondrial β-oxidation of fatty acids[34]; en-

Table 8-7: Effects of PPAR α Activation

- Suppresses the monocyte-macrophage poB-48 receptor[51]

- Inhibits basal and TGF-β-1 stimulated proliferation and proteoglycan production in human vascular smooth muscle cells[52]

- Limits the expression of proinflammatory cytokines, such as IFN-γ, in human T lymphocytes[53]

- Reduces vascular inflammation by repressing NF-κ B and AP-I transcriptional activity[54]

- Inhibits tissue factor and fibrinogen synthesis[54]

- Inhibits vascular endothelial growth factor receptor-2 expression[55]

- Improves endothelial dysfunction induced by Ang II[56]

- Down-regulates expression of NF-κ-B in lymphocytes[57]

- Up-regulates macrophage lipoprotein lipase[58]

- Inhibits expression of inflammatory genes, such as interleukin-6, cyclooxygenase-2, and endothelin-1[59]

- Inhibits expression of monocyte-recruiting proteins such as vascular cell adhesion molecule (VCAM)-1[59]

- Induces apoptosis in monocyte-derived macrophages[59]

- Reduces C-reactive protein

From Coban et al[60] and Despres et al[61]

hanced synthesis of apolipoprotein AI[35] and apolipoprotein AII[36]; modulation of apolipoprotein A5 synthesis[37]; down-regulation of apolipoprotein CIII synthesis[38]; inhibition of cholesterol[39] and bile acid synthesis[40]; and enhancement of biliary secretion of cholesterol.[41]

As a result of these actions, the fibrates have multiple effects on serum lipoprotein levels. The major actions include reduction of plasma TG by 25% to 50%[42]; reduction in apolipoprotein CIII-enriched remnant lipoproteins[43]; a variable reduction of LDL-cholesterol (depending on fibrate)[42,44,45]; transformation of smaller LDL into larger LDL particles[46]; and increase of HDL cholesterol.[47-49] Among fibrates, fenofibrate has the most LDL-lowering potential. The greatest reductions in HDL cholesterol are seen in patients with elevated TG.[50]

Effects of fibrates, inflammation, and atherogenic pathways. Recent research suggests that activation of PPAR α by fibrates can occur in nonhepatic tissues (or cells). This has led to speculation that some of the potentially beneficial effects of fibrates could be through direct action on atherogenic processes. Table 8-7 lists some effects of activation.

Many of the actions described in Table 8-7 could be antiatherogenic, but activation of PPAR α might be proatherogenic.[62] Therefore, the only real test of the efficacy of fibrates in reducing ASCVD risk must come through clinical trials.

Effects of fibrates on major coronary events. Several clinical trials have compared fibrates for coronary outcomes. Findings are summarized in Table 8-8. Although reductions in CHD end points varied from trial to trial, there was a strong overall trend toward reduction in events. These findings are reinforced by angiographic trials, which collectively show less progression of coronary lesions in patients treated with fibrates (compared to placebo) (Table 8-9).

Side effects of fibrates. The WHO clofibrate trial[63] suggests that clofibrate increases non-CHD mortality. This increase offsets any benefit from reduced CHD risk. Specific side effects were not identified in this trial. However, the findings impeded the use of fibrates for many years. Subsequent clinical trials have shown no increase in non-CHD mortality. Nonetheless, there are some side effects that must be recognized. These include GI distress, skin rashes, cholesterol gallstones, and myopathy. About 2% to 5% of patients treated with fibrates will develop cholesterol gallstones. Patients at risk for myopathy include those with end-stage renal disease and those taking statins. For the former, the dose of fibrates must be reduced according to the package insert for the drug. For concomitant use with statins, gemfibrozil should be avoided. The exceptionally high risk for myopathy with the combination of cerivastatin + gemfibrozil contributed to the removal of cerivastatin from the market.[74]

Whether used alone or combined with a statin, fibrates are not equivalent in their contribution to myopathy.[75,76] It appears that gemfibrozil interferes with statin catabolism, whereas fenofibrate does not.[77] Fenofibrate should therefore be less likely to induce myopathy in combination with statins than gemfibrozil. Fenofibrate also has the advantage of once-a-day dosing, and it is generally well tolerated.

Clinical use of fibrates in the metabolic syndrome. Fibrates are particularly useful in persons with very high TG levels (>500 mg/dL) to reduce the risk for acute pancreatitis. Fenofibrate apparently has an advantage of safety over gemfibrozil when used in combination with statins in patients with atherogenic dyslipidemia.[8] In patients with the metabolic syndrome, the primary goal of therapy is to achieve the LDL-cholesterol goal. The goal is determined by the risk status of the patient (Table 8-1). If the patient is above goal after lifestyle therapies, an LDL-lowering drug is indicated. The usual choice is a statin, although fenofibrate might be considered if the TG levels are relatively low. LDL lowering with fenofibrate is best when TG levels are low. The secondary target of therapy is non-

Table 8-8: Clinical Trials With CHD End Points Using Fibrate Therapy (Modified From ATP III Report)

Trial/Drug/ Duration of Intervention	Number of Subjects	Group
WHO trial[63] Clofibrate 5 yr	15,745 men from Edinburgh (subsets: n = 4,935)	Placebo On-treatment
Helsinki Heart Study[64] Gemfibrozil 5 yr	4,081 men	Baseline
Coronary Drug Project[65] Clofibrate 5 yr	1,103 men on clofibrate Treatment vs 2,789 placebo	Baseline On-treatment
Newcastle trial[66] Clofibrate 5 yr	400 men 97 women	Baseline On-treatment Baseline On-treatment
Scottish Trial[67] Clofibrate 6 yr	593 men 124 women	Baseline On-treatment Baseline On-treatment

TC = total cholesterol
TG = triglycerides
NS = not significant

Lipid and Lipoprotein Values

TC (mg/dL)	TG (mg/dL)	Non-HDL-C (mg/dL)	HDL-C (mg/dL)	% Change in Coronary Event Rate*
257	210	-	-	-20%
229	160	-	-	$P=0.05$
289	175	242	47	-34%
				$P<0.02$
250	177	-	-	-5%
234	149	-	-	NS
245	337	-	-	-49%
217	215	-	-	$P<0.01$
270	-	-	-	
229	-	-	-	
264	-	-	-	-44%
229	-	-	-	NS
280	-	-	-	
228	-	-	-	

* Drug group vs placebo group

(continued on next page)

Table 8-8: Clinical Trials With CHD End Points Using Fibrate Therapy (Modified From ATP III Report)
(continued)

Trial/Drug/ Duration of Intervention	Number of Subjects	Group
Stockholm Study[68] Clofibrate+ Nicotinic acid 5 yr	219 men 60 women lipoproteins on subset	Baseline On-treatment
VA-HIT trial[69] Gemfibrozil 5 yr	2,531 men	Baseline On-treatment
BIP[70] Bezafibrate 6 yr	2,825 men 265 women	Baseline On-treatment

VA-HIT = Veterans Affairs High-Density Lipoprotein Cholesterol Intervention Trial Group, BIP = Bezafibrate Infarction Prevention Study

LDL-cholesterol (or apo B), for which Table 8-1 lists goals of therapy. If TG levels remain elevated and HDL-cholesterol levels are reduced after achieving the goals for LDL, VLDL, and apo B with an LDL-lowering drug, a TG-lowering agent (eg, fenofibrate) can be considered.

Lipid and Lipoprotein Values

TC (mg/dL)	TG (mg/dL)	Non-HDL-C (mg/dL)	HDL-C (mg/dL)	% Change in Coronary Event Rate*
251	208	203	48	-36%
218	166	-	-	P<0.01
175	161	143	32	-22%
170	115	136	34	P<0.006
212	145	177	35	-9.4%
202	115	161	41	P=0.26

* Drug group vs placebo group

TC = total cholesterol

TG = triglycerides

An important but unresolved issue is whether fibrates reduce risk for ASCVD events independent of their effects on plasma lipids. The favorable outcome of the VA-HIT trial particularly suggests such an effect, perhaps by mitigating the proinflammatory state. Furthermore, sub-

Table 8-9: Clinical Trials With Angiographic End Points in Patients Treated With Fibrates (Modified From ATP III Report)

Trial/Drug/ Duration of Intervention	N	Group
BECAIT[71] Bezafibrate 600 mg 5 yr	92 men; 80% had mixed dyslipidemia	Baseline On-treatment
LOCAT[72] Gemfibrozil 1,200 mg 2-3 yr	395 men with low HDL, all s/p CABG	Baseline On-treatment
DAIS[73] Fenofibrate	305 men 113 women with type 2 diabetes	Baseline On-treatment

BECAIT = Bezafibrate Coronary Atherosclerosis Intervention Trial,
DAIS = Diabetes Atherosclerosis Intervention Study,
LOCAT = Lopid Coronary Angiography Trial

group analysis of the VA-HIT trial suggests that the best results with gemfibrozil were obtained in persons with characteristics of the metabolic syndrome (ie, hypertriglyceridemia, insulin resistance, and/or type 2 diabetes).[78,79] A similar result was obtained with gemfibrozil in the

Baseline and Rx Lipid and Lipoprotein Values

Total Chol	TG	LDL	HDL	Mean change, minimum lesion diameter (mm)*
266	216	180	34	-0.17 placebo,
229	159	173	37	-0.06 bezafibrate, $P<0.05$
199	146	139	31	-0.04 placebo,
186	92	130	38	-0.01 gemfibrozil, $P=0.009$
216	214	133	40	-0.06 placebo,
~194	~154	~125	~43	-0.01 gemfibrozil, $P<0.029$

*Lower numbers signify less progression of lesions.

TC = total cholesterol

TG = triglycerides

Helsinki Heart Study[80] and with bezafibrate in the Bezafibrate Infarction Prevention study.[70] If these results can be confirmed in studies with fenofibrate, the combination of statin and fenofibrate will be particularly attractive for patients with the metabolic syndrome.

Nicotinic Acid

Three forms of nicotinic acid are available: crystalline, sustained-release, and extended-release (Niaspan®).[1] Another preparation (Advicor®) combines extended-release niacin with lovastatin. Crystalline nicotinic acid is less expensive than the other types, but it must be taken 2 to 3 times per day and can cause unacceptable flushing. Sustained-release nicotinic acid generally does not cause flushing, but it is more likely to cause hepatotoxicity than the crystalline form. Niaspan® can be taken once a day and causes less flushing than crystalline nicotinic acid and less hepatotoxicity than sustained-release nicotinic acid. Crystalline and sustained-release nicotinic acid can be purchased over the counter or by prescription. Over-the-counter nicotinic acid is less expensive, but its purity cannot be assured. Niaspan® can be obtained only by prescription.

Effects on lipoprotein metabolism. Nicotinic acid, like fibrates, effectively lowers TG levels. Nicotinic acid also raises HDL-cholesterol levels[1] more than any other lipid-lowering drug. It also moderately lowers LDL levels. The mechanisms underlying these changes are not known. Nicotinic acid acutely suppresses release of nonesterified fatty acid (NEFA) from adipose tissue, but this change probably does not account for the drug's effect on lipoprotein metabolism. This effect is more likely secondary to metabolic changes in the liver.

Efficacy of nicotinic acid for reducing major coronary events. Limited clinical trial data indicate that nicotinic acid reduces the risk for major coronary events. The Coronary Drug Project (CDP)[65] was a secondary prevention trial in which nicotinic acid therapy reduced recurrence of CHD events by 25%. Long-term follow-up showed that patients who received nicotinic acid had a lower total mortality than did the placebo group. The Stockholm Ischemic Heart Disease Study[68] was another secondary prevention trial in which nicotinic acid was combined with clofibrate. In this trial, total CHD mortality was lowered by 36%. The greatest benefit was observed in the subgroup with higher TG levels. Several angiographic trials[1] revealed that combined drug therapy in which nicotinic acid was one of the agents reduced progression of coronary atherosclerosis compared to control groups.

Side effects of nicotinic acid. Side effects include flushing, itching, skin rashes, GI distress, hepatotoxicity, hyperuricemia, and hyperglycemia. Thus, some patients who receive nicotinic acid cannot tolerate it on a long-term basis.

Use of nicotinic acid in patients with the metabolic syndrome. For efficacy of lipid lowering, nicotinic acid is an attractive agent to use in combination with statins in persons with the metabolic syndrome. The combination mitigates all of the lipoprotein defects of atherogenic dyslipidemia: elevated levels of TGRLP, apo B, small LDL particles, and low HDL cholesterol. It is particularly efficacious for raising HDL levels. However, nicotinic acid can induce elevations of plasma glucose in some patients. Nicotinic acid can be used in patients with type 2 diabetes, but the dose should be kept low (1 to 2 g/d).[81] In persons with impaired glucose tolerance or impaired fasting glucose, any rise in plasma glucose can push the level above the threshold for categorical diabetes. These changes in glucose do not preclude the use of nicotinic acid in patients with the metabolic syndrome, but they make careful monitoring of glycemic status necessary.

When nicotinic acid is used in patients with the metabolic syndrome, several points of therapy should be remembered. If crystalline nicotinic acid is used, the initial dose should be very low (eg, 50 mg three times daily). The dose can then be doubled every 3 days up to about 1 g/d. The response in lipid and glucose levels should be rechecked. Further increments of 500 mg/d can be added, depending on lipid and glycemic status. In a patient with the metabolic syndrome, the dose generally should not exceed 2 g/d. Long-acting nicotinic acid is not recommended because of increased risk for side effects. Niaspan® can be initiated as a single dose at night. The initial dose should be 500 mg; it can be increased to 2 g/d, depending on lipid and glucose responses. In patients with type 2 diabetes, monitoring the glycemic response should include measurement of Hb A_{1c}.

References

1. Third Report of the National Cholesterol Education Program (NCEP) Expert Panel on Detection, Evaluation, and Treatment of High Blood Cholesterol in Adults (Adult Treatment Panel III) final report. *Circulation* 2002;106:3143-3421.

2. Grundy SM, Cleeman JI, Merz CN, et al: Implications of recent clinical trials for the National Cholesterol Education Program Adult Treatment Panel III guidelines. *Circulation* 2004;110:227-239.

3. Grundy SM: Low-density lipoprotein, non-high-density lipoprotein, and apolipoprotein B as targets of lipid-lowering therapy. *Circulation* 2002;106:2526-2529.

4. Heart Protection Study Collaborative Group: MRC/BHF Heart Protection Study of cholesterol lowering with simvastatin in 20,536 high-risk individuals: a randomised placebo-controlled trial. *Lancet* 2002;360:7-22.

5. Cannon CP, Braunwald E, McCabe CH, et al: Intensive versus moderate lipid lowering with statins after acute coronary syndromes. *N Engl J Med* 2004;350:1495-1504.

6. Nissen SE, Tuzcu EM, Schoenhagen P, et al: Effect of intensive compared with moderate lipid-lowering therapy on progression of coronary atherosclerosis: a randomized controlled trial. *JAMA* 2004;291:1071-1080.

7. de Lemos JA, Blazing MA, Wiviott SD, et al: Early intensive vs a delayed conservative simvastatin strategy in patients with acute coronary syndromes: phase Z of the A to Z trial. *JAMA* 2004;292:1307-1316.

8. Vega GL, Ma PT, Cater NB, et al: Effects of adding fenofibrate (200 mg/day) to simvastatin (10 mg/day) in patients with combined hyperlipidemia and metabolic syndrome. *Am J Cardiol* 2003;91:956-960.

9. Executive summary of the clinical guidelines on the identification, evaluation, and treatment of overweight and obesity in adults. *Arch Intern Med* 1998;158:1855-1867.

10. Clinical Guidelines on the Identification, Evaluation, and Treatment of Overweight and Obesity in Adults—The Evidence Report. National Institutes of Health. *Obes Res* 1998;(6 suppl 2):51S-209S.

11. Foster GD, Wyatt HR, Hill JO, et al: A randomized trial of a low-carbohydrate diet for obesity. *N Engl J Med* 2003;348:2082-2090.

12. Ballantyne CM, Olsson AG, Cook TJ, et al: Influence of low high-density lipoprotein cholesterol and elevated triglyceride on coronary heart disease events and response to simvastatin therapy in 4S. *Circulation* 2001;104:3046-3051.

13. Grundy SM: HMG-CoA reductase inhibitors for treatment of hypercholesterolemia. *N Engl J Med* 1988;319:24-33.

14. Endo A: The discovery and development of HMG CoA reductase inhibitors. *J Lipid Res* 1992;33:1569-1582.

15. Bocan TM: Pleiotropic effects of HMG-CoA reductase inhibitors. *Curr Opin Investig Drugs* 2002;3:1312-1317.

16. Shepherd J, Blauw GJ, Murphy MB, et al: Pravastatin in elderly individuals at risk of vascular disease (PROSPER): a randomised controlled trial. *Lancet* 2002;360:1623-1630.

17. Shepherd J, Cobbe SM, Ford I, et al: Prevention of coronary heart disease with pravastatin in men with hypercholesterolemia.West of Scotland Coronary Prevention Study Group. *N Engl J Med* 1995;333:1301-1307.

18. Downs JR, Clearfield M, Weis S, et al: Primary prevention of acute coronary events with lovastatin in men and women with average cholesterol levels: results of AFCAPS/TexCAPS. Air Force/Texas Coronary Atherosclerosis Prevention Study. *JAMA* 1998;279:1615-1622.

19. Sever PS, Dahlof B, Poulter NR, et al: Prevention of coronary and stroke events with atorvastatin in hypertensive patients who have average or lower-than-average cholesterol concentrations, in the Anglo-Scandinavian Cardiac Outcomes Trial—Lipid Lowering Arm (ASCOT-LLA): a multicentre randomised controlled trial. *Lancet* 2003;361:1149-1158.

20. Randomised trial of cholesterol lowering in 4444 patients with coronary heart disease: the Scandinavian Simvastatin Survival Study (4S). *Lancet* 1994;344:1383-1389.

21. Sacks FM, Pfeffer MA, Moye LA, et al: The effect of pravastatin on coronary events after myocardial infarction in patients with average cholesterol levels. Cholesterol and Recurrent Events Trial Investigators. *N Engl J Med* 1996;335:1001-1009.

22. Prevention of cardiovascular events and death with pravastatin in patients with coronary heart disease and a broad range of initial cholesterol levels. The Long-Term Intervention with Pravastatin in Ischaemic Disease (LIPID) Study Group. *N Engl J Med* 1998;339:1349-1357.

23. Grundy SM: Statin trials and goals of cholesterol-lowering therapy. *Circulation* 1998;97:1436-1439.

24. Pasternak RC, Smith SC Jr, Bairey-Merz CN, et al: ACC/AHA/NHLBI Clinical Advisory on the use and safety of statins. *Circulation* 2002;106:1024-1028.

25. Miettinen TA, Puska P, Gylling H, et al: Reduction of serum cholesterol with sitostanol-ester margarine in a mildly hypercholesterolemic population. *N Engl J Med* 1995;333:1308-1312.

26. Plat J, van Onselen EN, van Heugten MM, et al: Effects on serum lipids, lipoproteins and fat soluble antioxidant concentrations of consumption frequency of margarines and shortenings enriched with plant stanol esters. *Eur J Clin Nutr* 2000;54:671-677.

27. Ballantyne CM, Houri J, Notarbartolo A, et al: Effect of ezetimibe coadministered with atorvastatin in 628 patients with primary hypercholesterolemia: a prospective, randomized, double-blind trial. *Circulation* 2003;107:2409-2415.

28. Grundy SM: Alternative approaches to cholesterol-lowering therapy. *Am J Cardiol* 2002;90:1135-1138.

29. The Lipid Research Clinics Coronary Primary Prevention Trial Results: I. Reduction in the incidence of coronary heart disease. *JAMA* 1984;251:351-364.

30. Bays H, Dujovne C: Colesevelam HCl: a non-systemic lipid-altering drug. *Expert Opin Pharmacother* 2003;4:779-790.

31. Garg A, Grundy SM: Cholestyramine therapy for dyslipidemia in non-insulin-dependent diabetes mellitus. A short-term, double-blind, crossover trial. *Ann Intern Med* 1994;121:416-422.

32. Lee CH, Olson P, Evans RM: Minireview: lipid metabolism, metabolic diseases, and peroxisome proliferator-activated receptors. *Endocrinology* 2003;144:2201-2207.

33. Bremer J: The biochemistry of hypo- and hyperlipidemic fatty acid derivatives: metabolism and metabolic effects. *Prog Lipid Res* 2001;40:231-268.

34. Minnich A, Tian N, Byan L, et al: A potent PPAR alpha agonist stimulates mitochondrial fatty acid beta-oxidation in liver and skeletal muscle. *Am J Physiol Endocrinol Metab* 2001;280: E270-E279.

35. Vu-Dac N, Schoonjans K, Laine B, et al: Negative regulation of the human apolipoprotein A-I promoter by fibrates can be attenuated by the interaction of the peroxisome proliferator-activated receptor with its response element. *J Biol Chem* 1994;269: 31012-31018.

36. Vu-Dac N, Schoonjans K, Kosykh V, et al: Fibrates increase human apolipoprotein A-II expression through activation of the peroxisome proliferator-activated receptor. *J Clin Invest* 1995;96: 741-750.

37. Vu-Dac N, Gervois P, Jakel H, et al: Apolipoprotein A5, a crucial determinant of plasma triglyceride levels, is highly responsive to peroxisome proliferator-activated receptor alpha activators. *J Biol Chem* 2003;278:17982-17985.

38. Staels B, Vu-Dac N, Kosykh VA, et al: Fibrates downregulate apolipoprotein C-III expression independent of induction of peroxisomal acyl coenzyme A oxidase. A potential mechanism for the hypolipidemic action of fibrates. *J Clin Invest* 1995; 95:705-712.

39. Shiota Y, Ikeda M, Hashimoto F, et al: Effects of peroxisome proliferators gemfibrozil and clofibrate on syntheses of dolichol and cholesterol in rat liver. *J Biochem (Tokyo)* 2003;134: 197-202.

40. Post SM, Duez H, Gervois PP, et al: Fibrates suppress bile acid synthesis via peroxisome proliferator-activated receptor-alpha-mediated downregulation of cholesterol 7alpha-hydroxylase and sterol 27-hydroxylase expression. *Arterioscler Thromb Vasc Biol* 2001;21:1840-1845.

41. Grundy SM, Ahrens EH Jr, Salen G, et al: Mechanisms of action of clofibrate on cholesterol metabolism in patients with hyperlipidemia. *J Lipid Res* 1972;13:531-551.

42. Grundy SM, Vega GL: Fibric acids: effects on lipids and lipoprotein metabolism. *Am J Med* 1987;83:9-20.

43. Lemieux I, Salomon H, Despres JP: Contribution of apo CIII reduction to the greater effect of 12-week micronized fenofibrate than atorvastatin therapy on triglyceride levels and LDL size in dyslipidemic patients. *Ann Med* 2003;35:442-448.

44. Knopp RH, Brown WV, Dujovne CA, et al: Effects of fenofibrate on plasma lipoproteins in hypercholesterolemia and combined hyperlipidemia. *Am J Med* 1987;83:50-59.

45. Brown WV, Dujovne CA, Farquhar JW, et al: Effects of fenofibrate on plasma lipids. Double-blind, multicenter study in patients with type IIA or IIB hyperlipidemia. *Arteriosclerosis* 1986;6:670-678.

46. Eisenberg S, Gavish D, Oschry Y, et al: Abnormalities in very low, low and high density lipoproteins in hypertriglyceridemia. Reversal toward normal with bezafibrate treatment. *J Clin Invest* 1984;74:470-482.

47. Vega GL, Grundy SM: Comparison of lovastatin and gemfibrozil in normolipidemic patients with hypoalphalipoproteinemia. *JAMA* 1989;262:3148-3153.

48. Sasaki J, Yamamoto K, Ageta M: Effects of fenofibrate on high-density lipoprotein particle size in patients with hyperlipidemia: a randomized, double-blind, placebo-controlled, multicenter, crossover study. *Clin Ther* 2002;24:1614-1626.

49. Genest J Jr, Nguyen NH, Theroux P, et al: Effect of micronized fenofibrate on plasma lipoprotein levels and hemostatic parameters of hypertriglyceridemic patients with low levels of high-density lipoprotein cholesterol in the fed and fasted state. *J Cardiovasc Pharmacol* 2000;35:164-172.

50. Steinmetz A, Schwartz T, Hehnke U, et al: Multicenter comparison of micronized fenofibrate and simvastatin in patients with primary type IIA or IIb hyperlipoproteinemia. *J Cardiovasc Pharmacol* 1996;27:563-570.

51. Haraguchi G, Kobayashi Y, Brown ML, et al: PPAR(alpha) and PPAR(gamma) activators suppress the monocyte-macrophage poB-48 receptor. *J Lipid Res* 2003;44:1224-1231.

52. Nigro J, Dilley RJ, Little PJ: Differential effects of gemfibrozil on migration, proliferation and proteoglycan production in human vascular smooth muscle cells. *Atherosclerosis* 2002;162:119-129.

53. Marx N, Kehrle B, Kohlhammer K, et al: PPAR activators as antiinflammatory mediators in human T lymphocytes: implications

for atherosclerosis and transplantation-associated arteriosclerosis. *Circ Res* 2002;90:703-710.

54. Fruchart JC, Staels B, Duriez P: New concepts on the mechanism of action of fibrates and therapeutic prospectives in atherosclerosis. *Bull Acad Natl Med* 2001;185:63-74.

55. Meissner M, Stein M, Urbich C, et al: PPAR (alpha) activators inhibit vascular endothelial growth factor receptor-2 expression by repressing Sp1-dependent DNA binding and transactivation. *Circ Res* 2004;94:324-332.

56. Diep QN, Amiri F, Touyz RM, et al: PPAR alpha activator effects on Ang II-induced vascular oxidative stress and inflammation. *Hypertension* 2002;40:866-871.

57. Jones DC, Ding X, Daynes RA: Nuclear receptor peroxisome proliferator-activated receptor alpha (PPAR alpha) is expressed in resting murine lymphocytes. The PPAR alpha in T and B lymphocytes is both transactivation and transrepression competent. *J Biol Chem* 2002;277:6838-6845.

58. Li L, Beauchamp MC, Renier G: Peroxisome proliferator-activated receptor alpha and gamma agonists upregulate human macrophage lipoprotein lipase expression. *Atherosclerosis* 2002;165:101-110.

59. Neve BP, Fruchart JC, Staels B: Role of the peroxisome proliferator-activated receptors (PPAR) in atherosclerosis. *Biochem Pharmacol* 2000;60:1245-1250.

60. Coban E, Sari R: The effect of fenofibrate on the levels of high sensitivity C-reactive protein in dyslipidemic obese patients. *Endocr Res* 2004;30:343-349.

61. Despres JP, Lemieux I, Pascot A, et al: Gemfibrozil reduces plasma C-reactive protein levels in abdominally obese men with the atherogenic dyslipidemia of the metabolic syndrome. *Arterioscler Thromb Vasc Biol* 2003;23:702-703.

62. Molavi B, Rasouli N, Mehta JL: Peroxisome proliferator-activated receptor ligands as antiatherogenic agents: panacea or another Pandora's box? *J Cardiovasc Pharmacol Ther* 2002;7:1-8.

63. A co-operative trial in the primary prevention of ischemic heart disease using clofibrate. Report from the Committee of Principal Investigators. *Br Heart J* 1978;40:1069-1118.

64. Frick MH, Elo O, Haapa K, et al: Helsinki Heart Study: primary-prevention trial with gemfibrozil in middle-aged men

with dyslipidemia. Safety of treatment, changes in risk factors, and incidence of coronary heart disease. *N Engl J Med* 1987;317: 1237-1245.

65. Clofibrate and niacin in coronary heart disease. *JAMA* 1975; 231:360-381.

66. Group of Physicians of the Newcastle upon Tyne Region: Trial of clofibrate in the treatment of ischaemic heart disease. Five-year study by a group of physicians of the Newcastle upon Tyne region. *Br Med J* 1971;4:767-775.

67. Research Committee of the Scottish Society of Physicians: Ischaemic heart disease: a secondary prevention trial using clofibrate. *BMJ* 1971;4:7757-7784.

68. Carlson LA, Rosenhamer G: Reduction of mortality in the Stockholm Ischaemic Heart Disease Secondary Prevention Study by combined treatment with clofibrate and nicotinic acid. *Acta Med Scand* 1988;223:405-418.

69. Rubins HB, Robins SJ, Collins D, et al: Gemfibrozil for the secondary prevention of coronary heart disease in men with low levels of high-density lipoprotein cholesterol. Veterans Affairs High-Density Lipoprotein Cholesterol Intervention Trial Study Group. *N Engl J Med* 1999;341:410-418.

70. Secondary prevention by raising HDL cholesterol and reducing triglycerides in patients with coronary artery disease: the Bezafibrate Infarction Prevention (BIP) Study. *Circulation* 2000;102:21-27.

71. Ericsson CG, Hamsten A, Nilsson J, et al: Angiographic assessment of effects of bezafibrate on progression of coronary artery disease in young male postinfarction patients. *Lancet* 1996;347: 849-853.

72. Frick MH, Syvänne M, Nieminen MS, et al: Prevention of the angiographic progression of coronary and vein-graft atherosclerosis by gemfibrozil after coronary bypass surgery in men with low levels of HDL cholesterol. Lopid Coronary Angiography Trial (LOCAT) Study Group. *Circulation* 1997;96:2137-2143.

73. Effect of fenofibrate on progression of coronary-artery disease in type 2 diabetes: the Diabetes Atherosclerosis Intervention Study, a randomised study. *Lancet* 2001;357:905-910.

74. Staffa JA, Chang J, Green L: Cerivastatin and reports of fatal rhabdomyolysis. *N Engl J Med* 2002;346:539-540.

75.   Duell PB, Connor WE, Illingworth DR: Rhabdomyolysis after taking atorvastatin with gemfibrozil. *Am J Cardiol* 1998;81:368-369.

76.   Wierzbicki AS, Lumb PJ, Cheung J, et al: Fenofibrate plus simvastatin therapy versus simvastatin plus cholestyramine therapy for familial hypercholesterolemia. *QJM* 1997;90:631-634.

77.   Pan WJ, Gustavson LE, Achari R, et al: Lack of a clinically significant pharmacokinetic interaction between fenofibrate and pravastatin in healthy volunteers. *J Clin Pharmacol* 2000;40:316-323.

78.   Rubins HB, Robins SJ, Collins D, et al: Diabetes, plasma insulin, and cardiovascular disease: subgroup analysis from the Department of Veterans Affairs high-density lipoprotein intervention trial (VA-HIT). *Arch Intern Med* 2002;162:2597-2604.

79.   Robins SJ, Rubins HB, Faas FH, et al: Insulin resistance and cardiovascular events with low HDL cholesterol: the Veterans Affairs HDL Intervention Trial (VA-HIT). *Diabetes Care* 2003;26: 1513-1517.

80.   Tenkanen L, Manttari M, Manninen V: Some coronary risk factors related to the insulin resistance syndrome and treatment with gemfibrozil. Experience from the Helsinki Heart Study. *Circulation* 1995;92:1779-1785.

81.   Grundy SM, Vega GL, McGovern ME, et al: Efficacy, safety, and tolerability of once-daily niacin for the treatment of dyslipidemia associated with type 2 diabetes: results of the assessment of diabetes control and evaluation of the efficacy of niaspan trial. *Arch Intern Med* 2002;162:1568-1576.

Chapter 9

The Metabolic Syndrome and Type 2 Diabetes

Most people with type 2 diabetes have the metabolic syndrome in a more severe form. The metabolic syndrome is a heterogeneous condition consisting of several metabolic risk factors of varying severity. One risk factor is elevated plasma glucose, which, in its more severe forms, is called diabetes. Impairment of insulin secretion by pancreatic β cells also usually coexists with insulin resistance in clinically elevated glucose. In the presence of insulin resistance, the degree of glucose elevation depends largely on the severity of the defect in insulin secretion. This chapter examines the clinical approach to three levels of glucose elevation associated with the metabolic syndrome: impaired glucose tolerance (IGT), impaired fasting glucose (IFG), and categoric hyperglycemia (diabetes). IGT and IFG will be used synonymously with prediabetes.

Normoglycemic Metabolic Syndrome as a Risk Factor for Type 2 Diabetes

There are two concomitant causes of type 2 diabetes: insulin resistance and defective insulin secretion. Insulin resistance usually precedes the onset of defective insulin secretion by many years. Most people with the metabolic syndrome are insulin resistant, which makes their risk for ultimately developing type 2 diabetes approximately five-fold higher than that of people without the metabolic syndrome.[1] This higher risk exists even when the fasting glucose level is not elevated and glucose tolerance is normal. One of the major reasons for clinical detection of the metabolic syndrome is to identify patients who are at increased risk for developing type 2 diabetes.

First-line therapy for the metabolic syndrome is lifestyle change, primarily weight reduction and increased physical activity. The goal of lifestyle therapy is twofold: to reduce the risk for atherosclerotic cardiovascular disease (ASCVD) and to reduce the risk for type 2 diabetes. Drug therapies that target the metabolic risk factors may be required to prevent ASCVD. However, drug therapy is not indicated for prevention of type 2 diabetes when fasting and postprandial glucose levels are in the normal range.

Prediabetes: Impaired Glucose Tolerance/Impaired Fasting Glucose

Definitions

Prediabetes is defined either as a moderate elevation of fasting glucose (IFG) or as an exaggerated rise in plasma glucose during an oral glucose tolerance test (OGTT). The latter is IGT. IFG is defined as fasting plasma glucose in the range of 100 to 126 mg/dL,[2] confirmed by a second test, and IGT is defined as plasma glucose of 140 to 199 mg/dL 2 hours after oral administration of 75 g glucose.

The American Diabetes Association (ADA) recently lowered the threshold for IFG from 110 to 100 mg/d.[2] Although the pathophysiologic significance of IGT may differ from that of IFG, the prognostic significance with regard to ASCVD and type 2 diabetes seems to be similar.

The National Cholesterol Education Program Adult Treatment Panel III (ATP III)[3] set forth criteria for the metabolic syndrome that included IFG ($\geq$110 mg/dL) as one of the metabolic risk factors. The ADA's lower fasting plasma glucose cut point of 100 mg/dL is now accepted as an appropriate definition of IFG.[1] ATP III did not require oral glucose challenge to detect IGT; hence, it did not include IGT as a metabolic risk factor. The World Health Organization (WHO)[4] and the American Association of Clinical Endocrinologists (AACE)[5] accept IGT as a defining criterion for the metabolic syndrome, although neither explicitly defines the criteria for selection of patients for glucose testing.

Prediabetes as a Risk Condition

When IFG or IGT is identified in a normoglycemic person with other metabolic risk factors, the clinician should recognize an increased risk for type 2 diabetes and for ASCVD.

Risk for diabetes

The presence of either IFG or IGT carries an increased risk for development of diabetes. Presumably, most people who develop clinical diabetes will pass through a phase of prediabetes, either IFG or IGT or both. IFG and IGT predict new-onset diabetes similarly.[6] Many people with IFG have IGT, and vice versa. The concordance, however, is not perfect. For example, it has been claimed that elderly, less obese patients are more likely to manifest IGT, whereas IFG is more likely in obese patients.[7] An estimated 20% to 50% of people with IGT will develop type 2 diabetes over the next 10 years.[8] Presumably, the risk for diabetes is similar in persons with IFG.

Risk for cardiovascular disease

The relationship between IFG/IGT and ASCVD is complex. Because IFG is a common indicator of insulin resistance and the metabolic syndrome, it is unclear whether borderline glucose abnormalities are an independent risk factor for ASCVD. In the Framingham Heart Study, for example, IFG was not found to be an independent risk factor beyond the standard CVD risk factors.[1] Others have stated that IGT is an independent risk factor for ASCVD.[6] Whether this independence will stand up to rigorous multivariate analysis is not known.

Indications for Oral Glucose Tolerance Testing

Because the independent power of IGT to predict ASCVD is uncertain, the primary purpose of carrying out OGTT must be to identify people who are at risk for developing diabetes or who already have diabetes. Such identification would enable clinicians to prescribe interventions that could delay the onset or prevent the complications of diabetes. The cost and inconvenience of OGTT make it unsuitable as a routine measure, unlike the tests for plasma lipids or blood pressure. For these reasons, the ADA does not recommend routine OGTT. Fasting glucose measurements are preferred for detecting IFG or diabetes. However, some experts believe that OGTT should be performed in selected patients who might not be identified as being at risk for, or having, diabetes based on the results of fasting glucose measurements.[1] To date, no authoritative body has provided clear recommendations for OGTT. Suggested reasons to carry out OGTT include the presence of obesity or other metabolic factors (eg, ATP III-defined metabolic syndrome), diabetes in first-degree relatives, and a history of gestational diabetes. The question of whether to carry out OGTT in a particular patient must now be left to physician discretion.[1]

Therapeutic Reduction in Risk for Type 2 Diabetes

Therapeutic lifestyle changes

Mounting evidence indicates that lifestyle intervention at the stage of IGT/IFG or even normoglycemia can reduce the risk for developing type 2 diabetes in people with the metabolic syndrome. Several trials supporting the use of lifestyle intervention have been conducted in the past 20 years.[9-14] In general, weight reduction, improved diet, and increased physical activity were associated with improvements in metabolic risk factors, including insulin resistance.

The recent report of the United States Diabetes Prevention Program[15] provides additional support for the concept that the short-term risk for type 2 diabetes can be reduced through lifestyle change. This study randomized 3,234 patients with IGT/IFG to a placebo group or a treatment group given a diet and exercise regimen that achieved at least 7% weight loss and at least 150 minutes of physical activity per week. After 2.8 years of follow-up, new-onset diabetes was reduced in the treatment group by 58%.

Drug therapies

An important question in diabetes care is whether drug therapy should be used to prevent type 2 diabetes in higher-risk people. There are at least as many people with IGT/IFG as with type 2 diabetes, and many of those will progress to diabetes. In some populations, almost half of those with prediabetes progress to diabetes in 10 years. Although sustained reduction in weight and increased exercise will cut the risk of diabetes in half, successful lifestyle change is not common in routine clinical practice. Pharmacologic prevention is, therefore, an important issue.

The Diabetes Prevention Program[15] has demonstrated that metformin (Glucophage®) therapy will significantly reduce the risk for new-onset diabetes in patients with IGT/IFG. However, its findings raise several major questions. First, does delaying the onset of type 2 diabetes in patients with IGT/IFG modify their long-term prognosis? Second, is diabetes prevention cost-effective? The cost of this therapy per year of life saved has not been adequately evaluated. Third, can our health-care system afford the added burden of paying for diabetes prevention with drug therapy, even if it is medically worthwhile? Consider the following: if only 50% of patients with IGT/IFG will develop diabetes in 10 years, and if onset of diabetes is delayed in only 50% of these patients, then for every four people treated, only one will receive benefit. This number needed to treat is acceptable for the prevention of clinical CVD, but it may not be acceptable for a condition like type 2 diabetes, which is less of an immediate threat to life. Fourth, is drug therapy safe enough to justify its use? Metformin appears to be relatively safe. However, the long-term safety of thiazolidinediones (TZDs), which may be considered preventive therapy, has not been fully documented. Also, the costs of TZDs are a factor. Because these questions have not been adequately answered, current treatment recommendations do not support the use of drug therapies to prevent type 2 diabetes in people with IGT/IFG.

Type 2 Diabetes

Definitions

Guidelines for the classification and diagnosis of diabetes continue to evolve. Type 2 diabetes is a complex condition of which hyperglycemia is only one component. However, diabetes is conventionally equated with hyperglycemia.

If hyperglycemia is to be used as the defining parameter of type 2 diabetes, a clinical cutoff point must be determined. Two measures have been proposed: fasting hyperglycemia and postprandial hyperglycemia. The latter is typically determined by OGTT. The ADA does not recommend OGTT to diagnose diabetes and has adopted fasting hyperglycemia as the critical measure.

The defining level for the diagnosis of diabetes relates to the glucose level that will produce microvascular disease if maintained for a long period. In the past, a fasting plasma glucose level of >140 mg/dL was designated as the defining characteristic. Recently, the ADA lowered the threshold to >126 mg/dL.[2] Whether there is a significant difference between 126 mg/dL and 140 mg/dL in the risk for developing microvascular disease is not clear. The ADA's choice of fasting glucose as the defining parameter was influenced by the advantage of simplicity. Performing OGTT in patients who seem to be at risk for diabetes adds expense and inconvenience to routine clinical practice.

The WHO task force on diabetes classification favors the use of postprandial glucose levels for the diagnosis of diabetes.[4] The WHO cutoff point is a 2-hour glucose level >200 mg/dL. This approach adds time and expense to diagnosis but may more reliably identify people at risk for microvascular disease. However, it is not infallible; some patients with an abnormal OGTT will be normoglycemic or have only IFG on fasting samples. The major reason for recommending OGTT is that it allows earlier identification of diabetes and can lead to more aggressive risk reduction early in the course of the disease. The major drawbacks are the test's cost and inconvenience.

Goals of Therapy

The ultimate goal of therapy for type 2 diabetes is to prevent its complications. High on the list of complications are macrovascular and microvascular disease. Macrovascular disease takes the various forms of classic ASCVD, and prevention is achieved mainly by control of the risk factors for CVD, such as hyperglycemia, dyslipidemia, hypertension, and a prothrombotic state. Management of these risk factors will be addressed below. Microvascular complications include diabetic eye disease, chronic renal failure, and nephropathy. Control of elevated plasma glucose is paramount in preventing microvascular disease. The ADA publishes guidelines for glucose control.[16] Patients with type 2 diabetes should self-monitor their glucose levels. Fasting, preprandial, and bedtime glucose levels should be kept below 140 mg/dL. Ideally, fasting levels should be below 115 mg/dL. Hemoglobin A_{1c} levels should be maintained below 7%.

Treatment of Diabetes

A full examination of the treatment of type 2 diabetes is beyond the scope of this chapter. Nonetheless, a few general comments about treatment of diabetes in the context of the metabolic syndrome can be made.

Treatment of cardiovascular risk factors

Treating the risk factors associated with macrovascular disease, such as atherogenic dyslipidemia and hypertension, will reduce ASCVD risk in diabetic patients as well as in nondiabetic ones. Treatment with HMG-CoA reductase inhibitors (statins) significantly reduces risk for major ASCVD events.[17-19] Clinical trials further suggest that fibrate therapy to treat atherogenic dyslipidemia will decrease risk for ASCVD.[20,21]

Treatment of hypertension will improve prognosis for microvascular disease,[22] stroke,[23] and probably coronary heart disease. Aspirin therapy has not been shown specifically to reduce risk for ASCVD events in patients with diabetes, but its benefit for risk reduction in primary and secondary prevention in people without diabetes provides a strong rationale for using low-dose aspirin therapy in high-risk patients with type 2 diabetes. Ongoing clinical trials with antiplatelet drugs in patients with diabetes will provide more information on whether these drugs are effective in this population.

Therapeutic lifestyle changes

Many studies show that weight reduction and increased exercise improve glycemic control in patients with type 2 diabetes[24-26] and mitigate other metabolic risk factors.[27-29] Professional guidance on dietary and physical activity is an integral component in the management of patients with diabetes. The lifestyle approaches outlined in Chapter 6 for management of the metabolic syndrome can be applied to patients with type 2 diabetes. At the same time, it must be recognized that the risk for cardiovascular complications is high in these patients. Therefore, dietary changes alone are frequently inadequate to achieve desirable goals for hyperglycemia and other risk factors, and drug therapy is often required to supplement lifestyle changes.

Drug treatment of insulin resistance

Because insulin resistance contributes to hyperglycemia, the use of drugs to reduce insulin resistance may be considered. The TZDs are the major class of drugs available for this purpose. Their mechanism of action is not fully understood, although their primary target of therapy seems to be peroxisome-proliferator-activated receptor

(PPAR)-γ in adipose tissue, where they primarily reduce insulin resistance. In so doing, they decrease release of nonesterified fatty acids, dampen release of inflammatory cytokines and plasminogen activator inhibitor-1, and enhance adiponectin production.

The TZDs have proved useful for controlling hyperglycemia in many patients with type 2 diabetes. But despite their promise, they have some drawbacks that limit their use in clinical practice. They are relatively expensive. They cause edema in many patients and precipitate congestive heart failure in some,[30] most likely secondary to fluid retention. Finally, long-term therapy is often associated with weight gain not related to fluid retention. TZDs enhance the differentiation of adipose tissue, so the availability of more adipocytes may contribute to increasing obesity. Metabolic parameters are improved despite weight gain, but it remains to be seen whether weight gain with long-term use of TZDs will have detrimental side effects that offset the benefit.

An important but unresolved issue is whether a reduction in insulin resistance by TZDs will reduce risk for ASCVD. This may be the case if insulin resistance is at the heart of the metabolic syndrome. There are reports that use of TZDs reduces several of the metabolic risk factors.[31-35] If these changes truly translate into a significant risk reduction for ASCVD, TZDs could be recommended more strongly for therapy of type 2 diabetes. Ongoing clinical trials should provide valuable information on their efficacy for this purpose. Until these trials are completed, however, TZDs cannot be recommended specifically to treat type 2 diabetes.

Reduction in hepatic glucose output

Fasting hyperglycemia in patients with type 2 diabetes is mainly caused by increased gluconeogenesis and greater hepatic glucose output. One agent that targets this pathway is metformin. Clinical research shows that metformin therapy reduces hepatic glucose output. The mechanism for this favorable change is not known, but the general view is that the liver is the primary target of metformin action. A few reports suggest that metformin has systemic effects that reduce insulin resistance or improve insulin secretion.[36,37]

Metformin has many advantages as an agent to treat hyperglycemia,[38] including a history of generally safe long-term use in a widespread patient population. Moreover, it is relatively inexpensive and tends to cause some weight reduction by curbing the appetite. One drawback is that it can cause metabolic acidosis in patients with chronic renal failure. Most physicians will not use metformin when the serum creatinine is significantly elevated. Otherwise, the drug is generally well tolerated. An increasing number of physicians use metformin as the first oral agent in the treatment of hyperglycemia.

The United Kingdom Prospective Diabetes Study (UKPDS) raised the possibility that metformin reduces the risk for ASCVD in obese patients with diabetes.[39] Whether these suggestive findings will be confirmed in future clinical trials remains to be seen.

Therapy to enhance insulin secretion

The sulfonylureas have long been used to treat hyperglycemia of type 2 diabetes. Sulfonylureas are reported to stimulate insulin secretion by blocking ATP-sensitive potassium channels in the pancreatic β-cell membrane.[40] Because they are inexpensive, they often are used as first-line therapy. They can produce hypoglycemia, so their use must be monitored more closely than that of metformin. An alternative agent to sulfonylureas is nateglinide (Starlix®). This drug is a D-phenylalanine derivative that inhibits ATP-sensitive potassium channels in pancreatic β cells.[41] It also stimulates increased insulin secretion.

The concern that sulfonylureas could be cardiotoxic first arose in the University Group Diabetes Program (UGDP).[42] In the UGDP, treatment with the sulfonylurea tolbutamide (Orinase®) seemingly produced an increase in cardiovascular mortality. This was not confirmed in other clinical trials. The UKPDS[43] observed no indication of increased cardiovascular events or mortality with sulfonylurea treatment; if anything, there was a trend toward fewer myocardial infarctions. In theory, the sulfonylureas might adversely affect myocardial function because their mechanism of action could impair myocardial ischemic preconditioning. Some investigators suggest that some sulfonylureas are more likely to have adverse effects on the heart than other agents.[44] The potential cardiovascular dangers of sulfonylureas are unresolved.

Combined oral agents

Once diabetes develops, most patients show a gradual but progressive decline in insulin secretion. This phenomenon was clearly shown in the UKPDS. In clinical practice, therapy to reduce plasma glucose levels must be progressively intensified over time to maintain acceptable control. Standard practice is to add one oral agent to another for glucose control. The order in which oral agents are added varies according to the individual physician or to local practice. Some physicians start with an agent to enhance insulin secretion, whereas others start with metformin. Typically, TZDs are used last, if at all. A common problem in clinical practice is that therapeutic regimens lag behind the decline in insulin secretion. Consequently, control of hyperglycemia declines with time. Often, insulin therapy is initiated long after it should be. This period of inadequate control can be demonstrated by the presence of hemoglobin A_{1c} levels that are well above the recommended goal.

Insulin replacement and therapy

Eventually, oral hypoglycemic agents will prove insufficient to maintain recommended glucose control, and insulin therapy will be required in patients with type 2 diabetes. The indications for insulin therapy must be modified by clinical judgment. However, there are some general guidelines.[45] Foremost is the need to keep plasma glucose and hemoglobin A_{1c} within recommended ranges. Most authorities agree that insulin therapy is indicated when the hemoglobin A_{1c} level cannot be maintained below 8%. Others are more aggressive in initiating insulin (ie, at hemoglobin A_{1c} levels above 7%). Glycemic control can decompensate during infection, injury, or surgery in otherwise well-controlled patients. Insulin is required in patients who exhibit progressive weight loss from glucosuria or who develop ketosis in conjunction with severe hyperglycemia. Pregnancy and renal disease often are indications for use of insulin. Patients who cannot take oral hypoglycemic agents because of side effects should receive insulin.

There are many insulin therapy regimens. One approach is to continue oral hypoglycemic agents when starting insulin. Use of agents that reduce insulin resistance or lower hepatic glucose output along with insulin therapy is rational. However, with time, most physicians phase out oral agents along with the need for increasing insulin doses. There is considerable variability in use of hypoglycemia agents—oral and insulin—among different physicians. Fortunately, several forms of insulin are available, and these make it possible to tailor therapy to individual patients' needs.

References

1. Grundy SM, Brewer HB Jr, Cleeman JI, et al: Definition of metabolic syndrome: report of the National Heart, Lung, and Blood Institute/American Heart Association conference on scientific issues related to definition. *Circulation* 2004;109:433-438.

2. Genuth S, Alberti KG, Bennett P, et al: Follow-up report on the diagnosis of diabetes mellitus. The Expert Committee on the Diagnosis and Classification of Diabetes Mellitus. *Diabetes Care* 2003;26:3160-3167.

3. Third Report of the National Cholesterol Education Program (NCEP) Expert Panel on Detection, Evaluation, and Treatment of High Blood Cholesterol in Adults (Adult Treatment Panel III). Final report. *Circulation* 2002;106:3143-3421.

4.   Alberti KG, Zimmet PZ: Definition, diagnosis and classification of diabetes mellitus and its complications. Part 1: diagnosis and classification of diabetes mellitus: provisional report of a WHO consultation. *Diabet Med* 1998;15:539-553.

5.   Einhorn D, Reaven GM, Cobin RH, et al: American College of Endocrinology position statement on the insulin resistance syndrome. *Endocr Pract* 2003;9:237-252.

6.   Unwin N, Shaw J, Zimmet P, et al: Impaired glucose tolerance and impaired fasting glycaemia: the current status on definition and intervention. *Diabet Med* 2002;19:708-723.

7.   Qiao Q, Tuomilehto J: Diagnostic criteria of glucose intolerance and mortality. *Minerva Med* 2001;92:113-119.

8.   Alberti KG: Impaired glucose tolerance: what are the clinical implications? *Diabetes Res Clin Pract* 1998;40(suppl):S3-S8.

9.   O'Dea K: Marked improvement in carbohydrate and lipid metabolism in diabetic Australian aborigines after temporary reversion to traditional lifestyle. *Diabetes* 1984;33:596-603.

10.   Shintani TT, Hughes CK, Beckham S, et al: Obesity and cardiovascular risk intervention through the ad libitum feeding of traditional Hawaiian diet. *Am J Clin Nutr* 1991;53(6 suppl):1647S-1651S.

11.   Torjesen PA, Birkeland KI, Anderssen SA, et al: Lifestyle changes may reverse development of the insulin resistance syndrome. The Oslo Diet and Exercise Study: a randomized trial. *Diabetes Care* 1997;20:26-31.

12.   Eriksson KF, Lindgarde F: Prevention of type 2 (non-insulin-dependent) diabetes mellitus by diet and physical exercise. The 6-year Malmo feasibility study. *Diabetologia* 1991;34:891-898.

13.   Pan XR, Li GW, Hu YH, et al: Effects of diet and exercise in preventing NIDDM in people with impaired glucose tolerance. The Da Qing IGT and Diabetes Study. *Diabetes Care* 1997;20:537-544.

14.   Tuomilehto J, Lindstrom J, Eriksson JG, et al: Prevention of type 2 diabetes mellitus by changes in lifestyle among subjects with impaired glucose tolerance. *N Engl J Med* 2001;344:1343-1350.

15.   Knowler WC, Barrett-Connor E, Fowler SE, et al: Reduction in the incidence of type 2 diabetes with lifestyle intervention or metformin. *N Engl J Med* 2002;346:393-403.

16.   American Diabetes Association. Standards of medical care in diabetes. *Diabetes Care* 2004;27(suppl 1):S15-S35.

17.   Wilhelmsen L, Pyorala K, Wedel H, et al: Risk factors for a major coronary event after myocardial infarction in the Scandinavian Simvastatin Survival Study (4S). Impact of predicted risk on the benefit of cholesterol-lowering treatment. *Eur Heart J* 2001;22:1119-1127.

18.   Simes J, Furberg CD, Braunwald E, et al: Effects of pravastatin on mortality in patients with and without coronary heart disease across a broad range of cholesterol levels. The Prospective Pravastatin Pooling Project. *Eur Heart J* 2002;23:207-215.

19.   Migrino RQ, Topol EJ: A matter of life and death? The Heart Protection Study and protection of clinical trial participants. *Control Clin Trials* 2003;24:501-505.

20.   Robins SJ, Rubins HB, Faas FH, et al: Insulin resistance and cardiovascular events with low HDL cholesterol: the Veterans Affairs HDL Intervention Trial (VA-HIT). *Diabetes Care* 2003;26:1513-1517.

21.   Effect of fenofibrate on progression of coronary-artery disease in type 2 diabetes: the Diabetes Atherosclerosis Intervention Study, a randomised study. *Lancet* 2001;357:905-910.

22.   Adler AI, Stratton IM, Neil HA, et al: Association of systolic blood pressure with macrovascular and microvascular complications of type 2 diabetes (UKPDS 36): prospective observational study. *BMJ* 2000;321:412-419.

23.   Droste DW, Ritter MA, Dittrich R, et al: Arterial hypertension and ischaemic stroke. *Acta Neurol Scand* 2003;107:241-251.

24.   U.S. Department of Health and Human Services. Physical activity and health: a report of the Surgeon General. Atlanta, Georgia: U.S. Department of Health and Human Services, Centers for Disease Control and Prevention, National Center for Chronic Disease Prevention and Health Promotion, 1996, 278 pages.

25.   Zierath JR: Invited review: exercise training-induced changes in insulin signaling in skeletal muscle. *J Appl Physiol* 2002;93:773-781.

26.   Fletcher GF, Balady G, Blair SN, et al: Statement on exercise: benefits and recommendations for physical activity programs for all Americans. A statement for health professionals by the Committee on Exercise and Cardiac Rehabilitation of the Council on Clinical Cardiology, American Heart Association. *Circulation* 1996;94:857-862.

27.   Sacks FM, Svetkey LP, Vollmer WM, et al: Effects on blood pressure of reduced dietary sodium and the Dietary Approaches to

Stop Hypertension (DASH) diet. DASH-Sodium Collaborative Research Group. *N Engl J Med* 2001;344:3-10.

28. Appel LJ, Moore TJ, Obarzanek E, et al: A clinical trial of the effects of dietary patterns on blood pressure. DASH Collaborative Research Group. *N Engl J Med* 1997;336:1117-1124.

29. National Research Council. Diet and health: implications for reducing chronic disease risk. Washington, DC, National Academies Press, 1989:171-20.

30. Nesto RW, Bell D, Bonow RO, et al: Thiazolidinedione use, fluid retention, and congestive heart failure: a consensus statement from the American Heart Association and American Diabetes Association. October 7, 2003. *Circulation* 2003;108:2941-2948.

31. Olansky L, Marchetti A, Lau H: Multicenter retrospective assessment of thiazolidinedione monotherapy and combination therapy in patients with type 2 diabetes: comparative subgroup analyses of glycemic control and blood lipid levels. *Clin Ther* 2003; 25(suppl B):B64-B80.

32. Goldstein BJ: Current views on the mechanism of action of thiazolidinedione insulin sensitizers. *Diabetes Technol Ther* 1999;1: 267-275.

33. Yamada K, Kuzuya H, Nakano T: [Cardiovascular effects of the thiazolidinedione troglitazone.] *Nippon Rinsho* 2000;58:435-439. [Article in Japanese.]

34. Ginsberg H, Plutzky J, Sobel BE: A review of metabolic and cardiovascular effects of oral antidiabetic agents: beyond glucose-level lowering. *J Cardiovasc Risk* 1999;6:337-346.

35. Gouda BP, Asnani S, Fonseca VA: Effects of thiazolidinediones on cardiovascular risk factors. *Compr Ther* 2002;28:200-206.

36. Lupi R, Del Guerra S, Fierabracci V, et al: Lipotoxicity in human pancreatic islets and the protective effect of metformin. *Diabetes* 2002;51(suppl 1):S134-S137.

37. Patane G, Piro S, Rabuazzo AM, et al: Metformin restores insulin secretion altered by chronic exposure to free fatty acids or high glucose: a direct metformin effect on pancreatic beta-cells. *Diabetes* 2000;49:735-740.

38. Abbasi F, Chu JW, McLaughlin T, et al: Effect of metformin treatment on multiple cardiovascular disease risk factors in patients with type 2 diabetes mellitus. *Metabolism* 2004;53:159-164.

39.   Clarke P, Gray A, Adler A, et al: Cost-effectiveness analysis of intensive blood-glucose control with metformin in overweight patients with type II diabetes (UKPDS No. 51). *Diabetologia* 2001; 44:298-304.

40.   Ashcroft FM, Gribble FM: Tissue-specific effects of sulfonylureas: lessons from studies of cloned K(ATP) channels. *J Diabetes Complications* 2000;14:192-196.

41.   Dunn CJ, Faulds D: Nateglinide. *Drugs* 2000;60:607-615.

42.   Meinert CL, Knatterud GL, Prout TE, et al: A study of the effects of hypoglycemic agents on vascular complications in patients with adult-onset diabetes. II. Mortality results. *Diabetes* 1970;19(suppl):789-830.

43.   Intensive blood-glucose control with sulphonylureas or insulin compared with conventional treatment and risk of complications in patients with type 2 diabetes (UKPDS 33). UK Prospective Diabetes Study (UKPDS) Group. *Lancet* 1998;352:837-853.

44.   Riddle MC: Editorial: sulfonylureas differ in effects on ischemic preconditioning—is it time to retire glyburide? *J Clin Endocrinol Metab* 2003;88:528-530.

45.   Skyler JS: Insulin therapy in type II diabetes: who needs it, how much of it, and for how long? *Postgrad Med* 1997;101:85-90, 92-4, 96.

Chapter 10

Hypertension

All of the clinical criteria guidelines for the metabolic syndrome include elevated blood pressure (BP) as a component. The World Health Organization (WHO) report has defined elevated BP as a metabolic syndrome component as ≥140/≥90 mm Hg. The Third Report of the Expert Panel on Detection, Evaluation, and Treatment of High Blood Cholesterol in Adults (Adult Treatment Panel III [ATP III]) and the American Association of Clinical Endocrinologists have defined elevated BP associated with the metabolic syndrome to be ≥130/≥85 mm Hg. Furthermore, a patient being treated for hypertension can be assumed to have a metabolic risk factor.

The ATP III definition of elevated BP differs slightly from that of the recently released Seventh Report of the Joint National Committee on Prevention, Detection, Evaluation, and Treatment of High Blood Pressure (JNC 7) guidelines from the National Heart, Lung, and Blood Institute.[1] JNC 7 defines two categories of hypertension and adds a third, acknowledging the linear relationship between pressure and risk of atherosclerotic cardiovascular disease (ASCVD). This third category is called *prehypertension*, defined as a systolic blood pressure (SBP) of 120 to 139 mm Hg or a diastolic blood pressure (DBP) of 80 to 89 mm Hg. Eliminated from JNC 7 was a stage called *high-normal blood pressure* (SBP 130 to 139 mm Hg/DBP 85 to 89 mm Hg). ATP III identified the lower limits of high-normal BP as the threshold for elevated BP to define the metabolic syndrome.

Table 10-1: Blood Pressure Levels*

Classification	Systolic BP	Diastolic BP
Normal	<120	and <80
Prehypertension	120-139	or 80-89
Stage 1 hypertension	140-159	or 90-99
Stage 2 hypertension	>160	or >100

*Defined by JNC 7[1]

So far, the threshold for elevated BP in the metabolic syndrome has not been changed to 120/80 mm Hg, as might be suggested by new JNC 7 criteria. ATP III distinguishes between elevated BP and prehypertension. Thus, it seems inappropriate to call prehypertension a risk factor for the metabolic syndrome (Table 10-1).

Some hypertension investigators have been uneasy about including elevated BP as a risk factor for the metabolic syndrome for two reasons. First, the mechanistic interconnections between higher BP and other metabolic risk factors are not well understood. There is little doubt that hypertension has a multifactorial etiology; several of its causes may not even be metabolic. Second, several factor analysis reports of the metabolic syndrome fail to connect hypertension strongly with other risk factors.[2-9] This is not true for all studies, but the strength of the association between BP and other metabolic risk factors varies.

Despite these reservations, all major organizations that have recommended guidelines for the metabolic syndrome have included elevated BP as a component (see Chapter 6). The challenge for investigators is to explore more fully the mechanisms underlying hypertension and to relate them to the other metabolic risk factors.

Associations and Mechanisms of Elevated Blood Pressure

Although researchers cannot claim to have identified the fundamental causes of hypertension, an enormous body of information has accrued about factors associated with elevated BP. Among these, obesity ranks high. Several theories propose mechanisms to connect hypertension with obesity. One theory looks to appetite control and thermoregulation, where leptin provides the key link.[10,11] Others point to the release of excessive bioactive agents by adipose tissue. Another theory implicates sodium retention, perhaps from hyperinsulinemia, adipokines, or renal vascular changes. Still another suggests vasoconstriction induced by increased sympathetic activity.[12,13] Insulin resistance once held favor, with hyperinsulinemia being the mediator at the level of the kidney or sympathetic nervous system.[14] The role of hyperinsulinemia in causing hypertension, however, remains unproven.[15] Obesity probably is linked to higher BP through mechanisms known to regulate BP–the hormonal system, the sympathetic system, the mechanical properties of blood vessels, and control of intravascular volume.

Renin-Angiotensin-Aldosterone System

One key regulator of BP is the renin-angiotensin-aldosterone system (RAAS). Angiotensin II stimulates production of aldosterone, which in turn stimulates the kidneys to retain sodium, increasing intravascular volume. Angiotensin II directly increases vascular wall tension, and according to some investigators, it also increases production of reactive oxygen species, specifically superoxide, in human arteries.[16] This could promote oxidation of low-density lipoprotein (LDL), enhancing atherogenesis.

Sympathetic Nervous System

Sympathetic tone appears to be elevated in some people with hypertension. Several factors related to the metabolic syndrome may increase sympathetic tone, including insulin, leptin, nonesterified fatty acids, cytokines, triiodothyronine, eicosanoids, sleep apnea, nitric oxide (NO), endorphins, and neuropeptide Y.[17]

Intravascular Volume, Vascular Tone, and Compliance

Age-related stiffening of large arteries combined with accumulating atherosclerosis decreases vascular compliance, raising BP. This effect contributes substantially to systolic hypertension in older people. However, some investigators question whether this mechanism of hypertension relates to the metabolic syndrome.

Vascular Endothelium

Among the prohypertensive factors accompanying the metabolic syndrome are those adversely affecting vascular endothelium. The endothelium produces both vasodilators and vasoconstrictors. The former includes NO, prostacyclin, endothelium-derived hyperpolarizing factors, and C-type natriuretic peptide. Vasoconstrictors include endothelin-1 and cyclooxygenase products such as endoperoxides and thromboxanes, collectively known as endothelium-derived contracting factors. The endothelium also influences leukocytes, platelets, and blood coagulation[18] and is a major source of cytokines—particularly IL-6, a primary inflammatory stimulant.[19]

Patients with insulin resistance have elevated levels of insulin and insulin-like growth factor-1. Insulin itself appears to increase endothelial release of NO, a principal vasodilator, whereas insulin resistance may diminish this response.[20] Endothelial dysfunction has been implicated as an important factor in atherogenesis. Presumably, abnormalities in substances released by dysfunctional endothelium stimulate atherogenic processes in the subendothelium. Moreover, the normal barrier to influx of inflammatory cells into subendothelial spaces may be impaired when the endothelium is dysfunctional.

Clinical Complications of Hypertension
Cardiovascular Disease

Hypertension is a risk factor for every form of cardiovascular disease (CVD), including stroke, myocardial infarction (MI), heart failure, and chronic renal failure. Dozens of studies conclude that for individuals 40 to 70 years of age, each increment of 20 mm Hg in SBP or 10 mm Hg in DBP doubles the risk of ASCVD. This linear relationship extends across the entire BP range from 115/75 to 185/115 mm Hg.[21] The Framingham Heart Study further demonstrated that hypertension is more likely the older one gets. Individuals with a 'normal' BP at age 55 still carry a 90% lifetime risk for developing hypertension.[22] Treatment of hypertension, conversely, lowers risk for its complications. Antihypertensive therapy produces reductions in stroke incidence averaging 35% to 40%; MI, 20% to 25%; and heart failure, more than 50%.[23]

Proteinuria

Proteinuria is considered a metabolic dysfunction of renal glomeruli related to hypertension. Its presence carries predictive power for CVD events. This is true in hypertensive patients with and without diabetes.

Association of Hypertension With Type 2 Diabetes

Hypertension is strongly associated with type 2 diabetes and proportionally related to cardiovascular mortality in diabetic patients, as was discovered in the 347,978 men screened for the Multiple Risk Factor Intervention Trial[24] (Figure 10-1). When other components of the metabolic syndrome are added to hypertension, the risk is substantially increased (Figure 10-2). This linear increase demonstrates dramatically the intimate interrelationship among all the components, because which components are present appears to matter less than the combined synergistic influence of each additional one.

Benefits of Hypertension Treatment

JNC 7 reviewed benefits from treatment of hypertension as revealed by a large number of clinical trials.[1] For

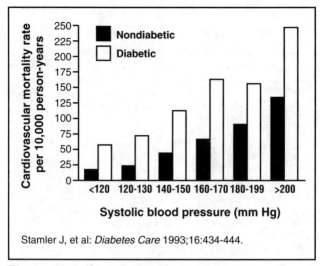

Stamler J, et al: *Diabetes Care* 1993;16:434-444.

Figure 10-1: Systolic blood pressure and cardiovascular mortality in type 2 diabetes.

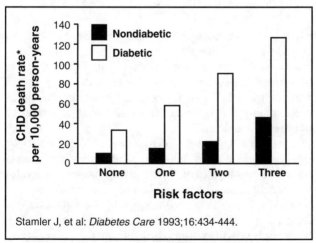

Stamler J, et al: *Diabetes Care* 1993;16:434-444.

Figure 10-2: Coronary heart disease (CHD) mortality according to risk-factor status.

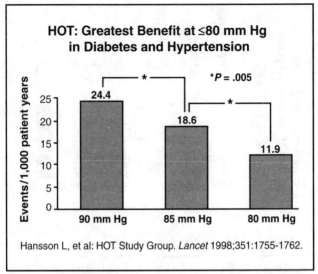

Figure 10-3: Hypertension Optimal Treatment (HOT) Study greatest benefit.

patients who have stage 1 hypertension (SBP 140 to 159 mm Hg and/or DBP 90 to 99 mm Hg) plus other CVD risk factors, achieving a sustained 12 mm Hg reduction in SBP over 10 years will prevent one death for every 11 patients treated. When CVD or target organ damage is present, only nine patients will require such BP reduction to prevent one death.[25]

Treatment of hypertension in patients with the metabolic syndrome undoubtedly reduces risk for cardiovascular complications of elevated BP. Perhaps the best evidence for this benefit comes from clinical trials in patients with diabetes, which is usually accompanied by the metabolic syndrome. For example, the United Kingdom Prospective Diabetes Study (UKPDS)[26] clearly demonstrated a benefit from BP reduction in type 2 diabetics that extended well into what was previously considered a 'normal' range.

Table 10-2: Summary of the HOPE Trial: Benefits of ACE Inhibition

- Combined primary cardiovascular outcome was reduced by 25%.

- Risk of MI was reduced by 22%.

- Risk of cardiovascular death was reduced by 37%.

- Total mortality was reduced by 24%.

- Risk of undergoing cardiac revascularization was reduced by 17%.

- Risk of nephropathy was reduced by 24%.

- Risk of stroke was reduced by 32%.

Likewise, the Systolic Hypertension in Europe (Syst-Eur) study and the Hypertension Optimal Treatment (HOT) Study Group (Figure 10-3) both found benefits from controlling BP in type 2 diabetes.[27] Compared to placebo, active treatment produced a 41% drop in overall mortality, a 70% drop in cardiovascular mortality, a 62% drop in all cardiovascular events, a 69% drop in stroke, and a 57% drop in all cardiac events. The HOT study found the greatest benefit to occur at a DBP <80 mm Hg.[28] There were 24.4 events per 1,000 patients at a DBP of 90 mm Hg, 18.6 events at a DBP of 85 mm Hg, and 11.9 events when DBP was reduced to 80 mm Hg or less. Syst-Eur studied nitrendipine vs placebo in 492 diabetic patients; HOT evaluated the difference between treating a DBP of 90 mm Hg vs 80 mm Hg using felodipine (Plendil®).

Among the many trials that proved the effectiveness of angiotensin-converting enzyme (ACE) inhibitors, the Heart Outcomes Prevention Evaluation Study (HOPE) trial[29] studied the effect of ramipril (Altace®) in 3,577 diabetic patients with at least one cardiovascular risk factor but no proteinuria and no heart failure. A summary of results is listed in Table 10-2. The cardiovascular benefit was greater than that attributable to the decrease in BP. The investigators concluded that ACE inhibitors yield a vasculoprotective and renoprotective effect for people with diabetes. ACE inhibitors proved efficacious in three other trials:

- Captopril (Capoten®) was compared with placebo in 207 insulin-dependent (type 1) diabetics with proteinuria. Captopril treatment was associated with a 50% reduction in the risk of the combined end points of death, dialysis, and transplantation. The addition of a diuretic was required to control BP in 75% of patients.[30]
- 583 patients with renal insufficiency caused by various disorders were treated with benazepril (Lotensin®) for 3 years. The primary end point was a doubling of the baseline serum creatine concentration or the need for dialysis. Benazepril reduced the risk of reaching these points by 53%.[31]
- In a 7-year study of 94 type 2 diabetics with normal BP and microalbuminuria, treatment with enalapril (Vasotec®) resulted in an absolute risk reduction of 42% for nephropathy.[32]

The Losartan Intervention for Endpoint (LIFE) study compared losartan (Cozaar®, Hyzaar®) with atenolol (Tenormin®) in more than 9,000 patients and in a subgroup of 1,195 patients with diabetes. The relative risk for the primary end point—a primary cardiovascular event (death, MI, or stroke)—favored losartan with a risk ratio of 0.87. For the diabetic subset, the risk ratio was even more favorable to losartan—0.76. The all-cause mortality also favored losartan, with a risk ratio in the diabetic subgroup of 0.61 ($P = 0.002$). In addition, new-onset diabetes was less frequent with losartan. The investigators concluded that losartan seems to confer benefits beyond reduction in BP.[33,34]

The Fosinopril Versus Amlodipine Cardiovascular Events Randomized Trial (FACET) included 380 Italian patients with hypertension and type 2 diabetes. Fosinopril (Monopril®) and amlodipine (Norvasc®) had similar effects on biochemical measures (cholesterol, high-density lipoprotein [HDL] cholesterol, glycosylated hemoglobin, fasting serum glucose, and plasma insulin), but, compared with patients receiving amlodipine, patients receiving fosinopril had a significantly lower risk of the combined outcome of acute MI, stroke, or hospitalized angina (14/189 vs 27/191; hazards ratio = 0.49).[35]

The Appropriate Blood Pressure Control in Diabetes (ABCD) study followed 470 hypertensive, type 2 diabetic patients without overt albuminuria on nisoldipine (Sular®) or enalapril for 5.3 years to compare the effect of intensive and less-intensive BP control on the microvascular complications of diabetes. The intensively treated group achieved an average BP of 132/78 mm Hg; the other group averaged 138/86 mm Hg. There was no difference between the two drugs or the two BP goals in stabilization of renal function. However, more intensive BP control decreased all-cause mortality. The incidence of fatal and nonfatal MIs, a secondary end point, was significantly ($P = 0.001$) higher among those receiving nisoldipine (n = 25) compared with those receiving enalapril (n = 5).[36]

The Captopril Prevention Project (CAPPP) studied 10,985 patients from Sweden and Finland to compare ACE inhibition with conventional therapy in preventing fatal and nonfatal MI, stroke, and other cardiovascular deaths in patients with hypertension. Cardiovascular mortality was lower with captopril than with conventional treatment (76 vs 95 events; relative risk 0.77, $P = 0.092$), but fatal and nonfatal stroke was more common with captopril (189 vs 148; relative risk 1.25; $P = 0.044$).[37]

These three studies—ABCD, FACET, and CAPPP—demonstrated the superiority of ACE inhibitors over alternative treatments in reducing the risk of acute MI (63% reduction, $P < 0.001$), cardiovascular events (51% reduction, $P < 0.001$), and all-cause mortality (62% reduction,

**Table 10-3: Nonpharmalogic Lifestyle
Changes to Treat Hypertension**

- Cessation of tobacco use has benefits that greatly exceed the lowering in cardiovascular risk. Chapter 6 lists 21 separate tobacco-related problems and cites the 29 diseases known to be related to tobacco.

- Weight loss, even 5%, benefits the metabolic syndrome.

- Dietary changes must include two elements: reduction of calories and a change to less atherogenic menu items.

- Physical exercise has benefits independent of its favorable effects on weight loss.

- Diet pills are briefly and marginally helpful in some patients, mostly to help get them started on dietary changes.

- Bariatric surgery is one approach for grossly obese patients who have failed every other weight loss intervention.

$P = 0.010$). In none of the trials did the ACE inhibitors demonstrate any advantage in preventing stroke.[38]

The Prospective Randomized Amlodipine Survival Evaluation (PRAISE)[39] followed 1,153 patients with NYHA class IIIb or IV heart failure for a median 14.5 months on amlodipine (a long-lasting dihydropyridine [DHP] calcium channel blocker [CCB]) or placebo. All patients were also taking ACE inhibitors, diuretics, and digitalis. The investigators concluded that amlodipine reduced pump failure and sudden deaths only in nonischemic heart failure patients. Ischemic heart failure did not benefit from amlodipine.

The African American Study of Kidney Disease and Hypertension (AASK) compared ramipril, an ACE inhibitor, with amlodipine, a DHP CCB, in African American patients with hypertension and renal insufficiency. Three years into the study, the ramipril group experienced sufficiently less decline in renal function to end the study. The authors recommended that DHP CCBs be used with caution in patients with renal insufficiency.[40]

Taken together, studies of diabetic patients with hypertension demonstrate a benefit over and above that seen in patients without diabetes. Moreover, the benefit extends well into what was considered a 'normal' range of BP readings.

Treatment of Elevated Blood Pressure

Lifestyle Changes

Chapter 7 covered nonpharmacologic interventions as therapeutic lifestyle changes, emphasizing their preeminence as first, safest, most necessary, and most effective interventions. Table 10-3 provides a brief summary.

Antihypertensive Drug Therapies

Trials of BP treatment have tested every hypertensive agent and nearly every combination available. A common finding of all trials is the need to use more than one drug. As Figure 10-4 shows, an average of three agents was used in the six studies.

Thiazides and Potassium Sparers

Thiazide diuretics have been the foundation of nearly every antihypertensive regimen and, with a single exception, have outperformed every other single drug-treatment regimen. The exception was the Second Australian National Blood Pressure trial, in which a regimen that began with an ACE inhibitor was slightly better than one starting with a diuretic. Nevertheless, diuretics are still underused in practice,[41] for two reasons. First, other medications are more heavily promoted by pharmaceutical companies. Second, concerns exist about the adverse effects of thiazides on lipids, glucose levels, and electrolytes.

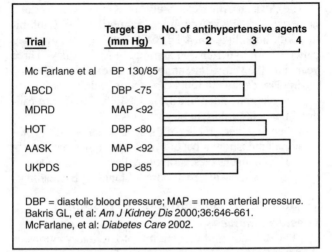

Trial	Target BP (mm Hg)	No. of antihypertensive agents
Mc Farlane et al	BP 130/85	
ABCD	DBP <75	
MDRD	MAP <92	
HOT	DBP <80	
AASK	MAP <92	
UKPDS	DBP <85	

DBP = diastolic blood pressure; MAP = mean arterial pressure.
Bakris GL, et al: *Am J Kidney Dis* 2000;36:646-661.
McFarlane, et al: *Diabetes Care* 2002.

Figure 10-4: Multiple antihypertensive agents needed to achieve target blood pressure in different trials.

Higher doses of thiazides raise triglyceride levels[42] and decrease insulin sensitivity.[43,44] The decrease in insulin sensitivity, probably mediated by hypokalemia,[45] has been nullified by adding potassium-sparing diuretics and has been shown to be of minor significance when lower doses are used (eg, 12.5 mg q.d. of hydrochlorothiazide [Dyazide®]).[41,45] The clinical significance of these effects is questionable in view of the substantial success thiazides have had in reducing end point events, even in patients who experience elevated lipid and glucose levels, especially when low doses are used.[46,47] However, clinical studies that have addressed this issue have been criticized for being too short in duration to encompass the long-term, deleterious effects of diabetes. Diabetes takes 2 decades to produce clinical cardiovascular disease. The Antihypertensive and Lipid-lowering Treatment to Prevent Heart Attack Trial (ALLHAT) followed patients for a mean of

5 years[48] and showed a significantly higher risk of new-onset diabetes with chlorthalidone (Clorpres™, 43% to 65%) than with amlodipine (30%) or lisinopril (Zestril®,18%).[49] Using thiazides as treatment for hypertension may generate excessive complications from diabetes later. JNC 7 still recommends thiazides as first-line therapy for hypertension. However, it is prudent to keep the dose relatively low and to monitor potassium levels, although it is unclear if potassium sparing will help avoid diabetes complications.

Thiazides have the additional benefit of reducing calcium loss from bone, thereby ameliorating osteoporosis.

The additional benefits provided by adding potassium-sparing agents to diuretics were originally thought to be limited to the potentiation of diuresis and the prevention of hypokalemia. When the link between hypokalemia and insulin resistance was recognized, the beneficial value of these agents was magnified. But it was not until a study was published in 1999 that the full benefits of spironolactone (Aldactone®) became evident. This article reported the early termination of the Randomized Aldactone Evaluation Study (RALES), not for the usual reason—adverse drug side effects—but because the results were so strongly positive that the investigators felt it was unethical to withhold the treatment from the placebo group. All 1,663 patients had severe heart failure and a left-ventricular ejection fraction of no more than 35%. All were taking an ACE inhibitor and a loop diuretic; most were taking digoxin. The active treatment group received 25 mg of spironolactone daily in addition to the other medications. After a mean follow-up period of 24 months, the spironolactone group experienced a 30% reduction in the risk of death both from sudden cardiac death and death from progressive heart failure, a 35% reduction in the frequency of hospitalization for worsening heart failure, and a significant improvement in the symptoms of heart failure.[50]

Hypokalemia (serum potassium <3.4 mmol/L) occurred in 10% of placebo-treated patients and in 0.5% of the spironolactone group. Hyperkalemia (serum potassium ≥5.5 mmol/L) occurred in 5% of the placebo group and 13% of the group taking 25 mg of spironolactone daily. Predictors of hyperkalemia included the use of ACE inhibitors other than captopril and baseline elevations of serum creatinine or potassium.[51]

Spironolactone has been reported to promote magnesium and potassium retention, increase uptake of myocardial norepinephrine, and attenuate formation of myocardial fibrosis. These effects are the result of counteracting aldosterone's inhibition of catecholamine reuptake, enhancement of potassium and magnesium excretion, and promotion of ventricular arrhythmias, myocardial fibrosis, endothelial cell dysfunction, and baroreceptor dysfunction.[52]

A recently released alternative to spironolactone is eplerenone (Inspra™), which has shown efficacy when given as an adjunct to angiotensin II receptor blocker (ARB) therapy and has proved its usefulness in heart failure in the Eplerenone Post-MI Heart Failure Efficacy and Survival Study (EPHESUS), causing fewer side effects (especially in men) than spironolactone.[53]

Furthermore, potassium sparing is hazardous in only a few conditions. Patients with impaired renal potassium clearance and those with a baseline potassium level >5.0 mEq/L are at greater risk from these agents.

Renin-Angiotensin-Aldosterone System Blockade

Among the multiple classes of agents available for treating hypertension, ACE inhibitors and ARBs uniquely slow the progress of diabetic nephropathy and reduce albuminuria.[30,54,55] The Reduction of Endpoints in NIDDM with the Angiotensin II Antagonist Losartan (RENAAL) trial has shown that treatment with losartan substantially reduces the incidence of end-stage renal disease.[56] Additionally, in more than 30 trials involving more than 7,000 patients with left-ventricular systolic failure, ACE inhibitors, when combined with diuretics, have proved their value by increasing survival, with an average risk reduction of 35% for the combined end points of mortality and hospitalization for heart failure.[57] This is because in addition to reducing systemic BP, angiotensin blockade dilates glomerular afferent arterioles, reducing glomerular capillary pressure; reduces inflammation by inhibiting monocyte/macrophage infiltration and oxidative stress; and reduces transforming growth factor-α induced collagen synthesis.[58,59] Angiotensin II induces superoxide, and therefore, agents that inhibit this hormone will reduce the action of these free radicals. ARBs have been shown to decrease plasminogen activator inhibitor-1 (PAI-1) levels and, as a result, slow and even induce regression of glomerular and vascular sclerosis.[60]

The choice between ACE inhibitors and ARBs depends on cost and the physician's greater experience with ACE inhibitors. ARBs are recommended primarily for patients who do not tolerate ACE inhibitors, usually because of the dry cough that is a common side effect. Theoretic differences exist between the two classes of agents. ACE inhibitors prevent the conversion of angiotensin to an active form, while ARBs allow angiotensin to be activated but prevent it from acting on specific target tissues. This may become important because angiotensin has effects that are not blocked by ARBs and generation pathways that bypass angiotensinogen conversion. Further research will uncover these effects and their clinical significance, if any.

The Valsartan Heart Failure Trial (Val-Heft) has warned of an antagonistic effect when ACE inhibitors and ARBs are used together. When added to prescribed therapy, valsartan (Diovan®) significantly reduces the combined end point of mortality and morbidity and improves clinical signs and symptoms in patients with heart failure. But patients taking valsartan and an ACE inhibitor did substantially worse than those taking valsartan alone. Those taking both experienced a 2.1% reduction in adverse cardiac events compared with those taking valsartan alone, who reduced their events by 13.1% (both results compared with placebo).[61] Further meta-analyses of several clinical trials that included the combination of an ACE inhibitor with an ARB have reached different conclusions. One[62,63] concluded that an ARB combined with an ACE inhibitor may benefit heart failure patients who are receiving all other recommended therapies, while another[64] limited its recommendation to patients not on β-blockers.

Another issue has recently surfaced about modulating the RAAS system—its potential to delay the onset of type 2 diabetes. One review[65] gathered all the clinical studies that reported a relationship between BP treatment and type 2 diabetes and tentatively concluded that data from the highest quality studies suggest that diabetes incidence is unchanged or increased by thiazide diuretics and β-blockers and unchanged or decreased by ACE inhibitors, CCBs, and ARBs.

$α_1$-Blockers

The $α_1$-blockers include doxazosin (Cardura®), prazosin (Minipress®), and terazosin (Hytrin®). $α_1$-Blockers improve insulin sensitivity and dyslipidemia[66]; however, they seem to be less effective than other antihypertensive agents in reducing cardiovascular events. In the ALLHAT study,[67] doxazosin exhibited a higher incidence of stroke, heart failure, and combined cardiovascular events compared to a thiazide. For this reason, the doxazosin arm of ALLHAT was discontinued prematurely. Although there may be indications for the use of $α_1$-blockers in combination with other antihypertensive drugs in more severe forms of hypertension, the use of $α_1$-blockers has largely been relegated to second or third choices.

β-Blockers Without $β_2$-Agonism

Many β-blockers are not $β_2$-agonists. These agents include atenolol, betaxolol (Kerlone®), bisoprolol (Zebeta®), metoprolol (Lopressor®), extended-release metoprolol (Toprol XL®), nadolol (Corgard®), propranolol (Inderal®), long-acting propranolol (Inderal® LA), and timolol (Blocadren®)

and can be divided into selective β_1-blockers and nonselective β_1- and β_2-blockers. Among the former, atenolol and metoprolol are the most widely used and are considered preferable because they induce less bronchial constriction and vasoconstriction. β_1 Blockade slows the heart rate, weakens heart contractions, and decreases RAAS activity.[68]

β-Blockers have been available for many years and have been proven to reduce MI and stroke. They are inexpensive, available as generics, and come in once-daily dose formulations (atenolol and extended-release metoprolol). JNC 7 recommends them as first-line treatment for patients without diabetes who have hypertension or previous coronary syndromes.[1] They carry a variety of side effects: fatigue, sexual dysfunction, cold extremities, depression, weight gain, negative inotropy and chronotropy, and asthma. Additionally, the suppressive effects of β-blockers on cardiac function may threaten an already marginal blood supply to other organs in patients with peripheral vascular disease.

The β_1-selective blocking agents, such as metoprolol and atenolol, have been reported to produce increased insulin resistance associated with increased fasting values of insulin and glucose. They may also suppress insulin secretion. These changes are associated with some increase in serum triglycerides and decreases in HDL cholesterol. Consequently, in theory, β_1-selective β-blockers are not desirable agents to use in patients with the metabolic syndrome.

Of concern for patients with the metabolic syndrome is the action of β-blockers to increase insulin resistance and to mask the BP changes and tachycardia that announce an episode of hypoglycemia, a fairly rare event in type 2 diabetes. However, other symptoms of hypoglycemia, such as dizziness and sweating, still occur.[69] Despite concern about the use of β-blockers in patients with diabetes, the UKPDS demonstrated that a β-blocker was just as effective as an ACE inhibitor in reducing microvascular disease in patients with type 2 diabetes.[70]

β-*Blockers With* β$_2$-*Agonism*

β$_2$-Agonist β-blockers include acebutolol (Sectral®), penbutolol (Levatol®), and pindolol (Visken®). These agents are nonselective β-adrenergic blockers that have partial agonist action at vascular β$_2$ receptors. They have been approved for the treatment of systemic hypertension. They have fewer adverse effects on glucose tolerance and serum lipoprotein profile than β-blockers without sympathomimetic activity. Because of the more favorable metabolic effects of these agents compared to β$_1$-selective β-blockers, they should be more desirable for use in treatment of hypertension in patients with the metabolic syndrome.

β-*Blockers With* α$_1$ *Blockade*

This class contains carvedilol (Coreg®) and labetalol (Normodyne®, Trandate®). Carvedilol has received increased attention recently because of its apparent benefit in the treatment of congestive heart failure. It is a nonselective β-adrenoreceptor antagonist combined with an α$_1$-adrenoreceptor antagonist. It is devoid of intrinsic sympathomimetic activity. Studies have shown that carvedilol causes fewer negative chronotropic and inotropic effects when compared with other nonselective β-blockers such as propranolol. Because it is a peripheral vasodilator, it seemingly improves renal blood flow more than nonselective β-blockers. Carvedilol may have other beneficial effects such as calcium channel blocking and antioxidant properties.

One potential advantage of carvedilol over other nonselective and selective β-blockers is that it appears to have fewer adverse metabolic effects. The metabolic changes of carvedilol were compared to those of metoprolol in the Glycemic Effects in Diabetes Mellitus: Carvedilol-Metoprolol Comparison in Hypertensives (GEMINI) study.[71] GEMINI was a randomized, double-blind study to compare the effects of carvedilol and metoprolol on glycemic control in 1,235 subjects 36 to 85 years of age with elevated blood pressure (>130/80 mm Hg) and type 2 diabetes. It was designed to study patients with diabetes and hypertension who were already being treated with an ACE inhibitor or an ARB and whose blood pressure was not controlled. If needed for BP control, open-label hydrochlorothiazide and a dihydropyridine calcium antagonist were allowed in the study. Both carvedilol and metoprolol were given in divided doses daily and were added to ACE inhibitor or ARB therapy. The primary end point of the study was the difference between groups and mean change from baseline hemoglobin A_{1c}. Other measures included the effects of the two drugs on fasting insulin levels, HOMA-IR, BP, and plasma lipids. Throughout the trial, carvedilol and metoprolol were well tolerated.

The changes in hemoglobin A_{1c} longitudinally throughout the study are shown in Figure 10-5.[71] Changes in other parameters are compared in Table 10-4.[71] The mean hemoglobin A_{1c} was increased on metoprolol but was unchanged on carvedilol (Figure 10-5). Other metabolic changes generally were more favorable on carvedilol than on metoprolol[71] (Table 10-4). BP changes were similar for the two drugs. Insulin resistance was significantly improved on carvedilol compared to metoprolol.[71] Moreover, progression to microalbuminuria with carvedilol was reduced to 47% of that with metoprolol.[71]

In summary, carvedilol did not worsen metabolic control in patients with type 2 diabetes, but a worsening was observed for those treated with metoprolol.[71] This study has implications for treatment of patients with the metabolic syndrome. In patients with impaired fasting glucose or impaired glucose tolerance, the use of usual β-blockers such as metoprolol can cause a worsening of glucose tolerance, causing some patients to cross the glycemic threshold for type 2 diabetes. In addition, for patients with type 2 diabetes, metoprolol and related agents can cause a worsening of glycemic control. The fact that carvedilol does not have this adverse effect appears to be a distinct advantage for treatment of hypertension in patients with the metabolic syndrome and with or without type 2 diabetes.[71]

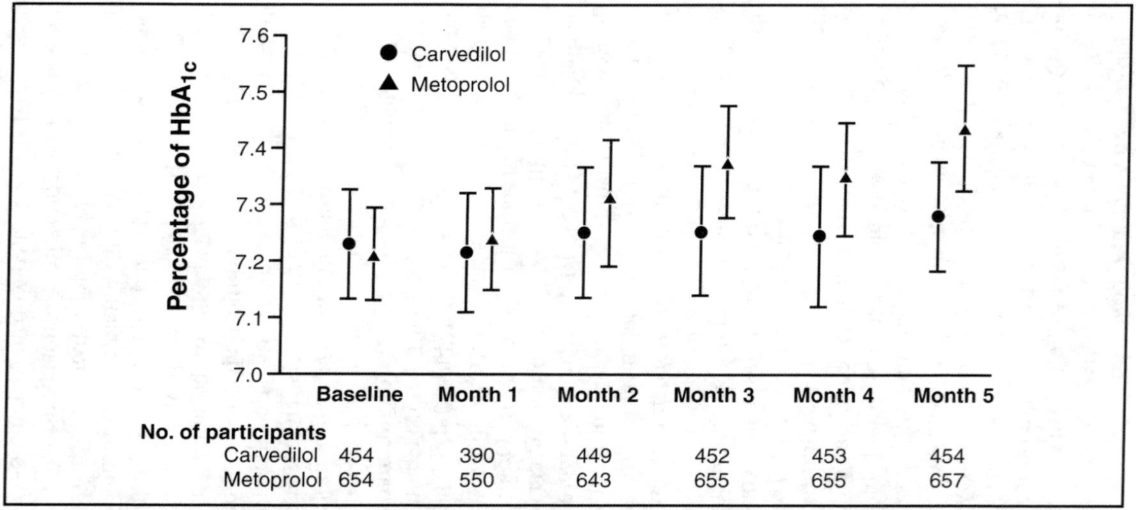

Figure 10-5: Glycosylated hemoglobin A$_{1c}$ at baseline and each maintenance month by treatment in the modified intention-to-treat population. The change from baseline to maintenance month 5 (primary outcome) was significant (mean difference [SD], 0.13% [0.05%]; 95% confidence interval, -0.22% to -0.04%; P=.004). Error bars indicate SD from mean. Bakris et al,[71] used with permission.

Table 10-4: Cardiovascular and Metabolic Measures in the GEMINI Study*

Parameter	Carvedilol (n = 454) % Change	Metoprolol (n = 657) % Change
Systolic blood pressure	-17.9 (0.7)	-16.9
Diastolic blood pressure	-10.0 (0.4)	-10.3
Mean heart rate	-6.7 (0.4)	- 8.3
ACR**	-14.0	+2.5
HOMA-IR†	-9.1	-2.0
Plasma glucose	+6.6	+10.6
Serum albumin	-19.4	-15.1
Body weight	+0.17	+1.2
Total cholesterol	-3.3	-0.4
LDL cholesterol	-4.4	-2.7
HDL cholesterol	-5.5	-5.7
Triglycerides	+2.2	+13.2

*Modified intention-to-treat analysis

**Urinary albumin/creatinine ratio

†Homeostatic Model Assessment—Insulin Resistance

Adapted from Bakris et al,[71] used with permission.

Calcium Channel Blockers

CCBs are commonly used because of their dual indications (hypertension and angina) and their low cost. CCBs, along with diuretics, appear to be more efficacious in African Americans, whose generally more severe hypertension responds less to monotherapy with β-blockers, ACE inhibitors, or ARBs. Combination therapy, as well as adequate diuresis, overcomes this discrepancy, but ACE inhibitor-induced angioedema occurs 2 to 4 times more frequently in African Americans.[72]

The primary difference between the two types of CCBs—nondihydropyridines (verapamil [Calan®] and diltiazem [Cardizem®]) and dihydropyridines (all the rest)—is their effect on cardiac conduction. The nondihydropyridines slow cardiac conduction and are more likely to cause serious arrhythmias. There are also major differences in the pharmacokinetics among the dozen-or-so agents available. Short-acting agents such as nifedipine (Procardia®) have been reported to increase the incidence of coronary events.[73,74] Longer-lasting agents such as amlodipine therefore are recommended for treating hypertension.

Combination Therapies

In an effort to simplify dosing and improve compliance, pharmaceutical companies have developed an assortment of oral medications that combine agents that are commonly used together. An example is a antihypertensive/diuretic agent. Other examples include birth-control pills, antidiabetic agents, and synergistic antibiotics.

Now a combination agent has been introduced for the metabolic syndrome that addresses two of its components in a single pill. Amlodipine, a CCB, and atorvastatin, an HMG CoA reductase inhibitor, are available together in eight different strengths (Caduet®). Several studies have suggested efficacy of this combination, such as in improving nitric oxide release and endothelial function,[75] retarding progression of coronary atherosclerosis,[76] and improving arterial compliance.[77]

We can look forward to more innovative combinations as disease associations and drug synergisms become increasingly recognized.

Summary

There are several considerations when setting priorities for introduction of drug therapy for hypertension in patients with the metabolic syndrome and type 2 diabetes (Table 10-5). The available evidence suggests that ACE inhibitors or ARBs should be first-line therapy. These drugs have been shown to slow progression of diabetic nephropathy and may have antiatherogenic properties. Although JNC 7 does not recommend specific antihypertensive agents for patients with diabetes, it lists thiazide diuretics as first-line therapy because of their low cost and evidence of efficacy in reducing stroke and MI in ALLHAT and other trials. However, as shown in ALLHAT, thiazides have the potential to worsen glucose intolerance. For this reason, they should be used in the lowest effective dose, and patients should be monitored for development of hypokalemia. Thiazides are not contraindicated in patients with metabolic syndrome with or without type 2 diabetes, but their potential side effects associated with these conditions should be kept in mind.

The usual selective and nonselective β-blockers used for treatment of hypertension may worsen glucose intolerance and atherogenic dyslipidemia. However, β-blockers that block α_1 and β receptors, such as carvedilol, are promising for treatment of hypertension in patients with metabolic syndrome and diabetes. Although metoprolol's ability to reduce risk for microvascular complications was shown to be equal to that of an ACE inhibitor in the UKPDS, the GEMINI study showed that carvedilol gave a better profile for glucose intolerance and dyslipidemia than metoprolol. The GEMINI study thus would favor carvedilol over metoprolol in treatment of hypertension in patients with the metabolic syndrome and type 2 diabetes.

Calcium blockers do not have adverse effects on metabolic parameters and thus can be used in a multidrug regimen for treatment of hypertension in the presence of glucose intolerance or diabetes. α_1-Blockers likewise

Table 10-5: Considerations for Choice of Antihypertensive Drugs in Patients With the Metabolic Syndrome and Type 2 Diabetes

Agent	Comments
Thiazide diuretics	• Inexpensive; JNC 7 first-line drug • Increased diabetes incidence in ALLHAT • Glucose intolerance worsened by hypokalemia
Potassium-sparing diuretics	• May reduce incidence of hypokalemia with thiazides • Can induce hyperkalemia with angiotensin-converting enzyme (ACE) inhibitors in patients with diabetes
β-Blockers ($\beta_1 \pm \beta_2$ blockers)	• Can worsen glucose intolerance in patients with impaired fasting glucose/impaired glucose tolerance or type 2 diabetes • Can raise serum triglycerides and reduce high-density lipoprotein • Reduce microvascular end points similarly to ACE inhibitor in UKPDS patients
β-Blockers with sympathomimetic activity (β_1, β_2 blocker + β_2 agonist)	Less worsening of glucose tolerance and fewer adverse effects on lipid profiles compared to β-blockers without sympathomimetic activity

ALLHAT = Antihypertensive and Lipid-lowering Treatment to Prevent Heart Attack Trial

Agent	Comments
Combined α- and β-blockers ($\beta_1 \pm \beta_2$ blockers + α_1-blocker)	• No adverse effect on glucose tolerance or serum lipoprotein profile • Metabolically superior to pure β-blockers (GEMINI)
ACE inhibitors and angiotensin receptor blockers	• No adverse effect on glucose tolerance or serum lipoprotein profile • Improve clinical outcomes in patients with chronic renal failure (with or without diabetes) • May be superior to other antihypertensive agents in secondary prevention to reduce atherosclerotic cardiovascular disease events
Calcium blockers	No adverse metabolic effects
α_1-Blockers	• Improves glucose and lipid profiles • Less effective on stroke, heart failure, and cardiovascular disease outcomes than thiazide diuretics (ALLHAT)

GEMINI = Glycemic Effects in Diabetes Mellitus: Carvedilol-Metoprolol Comparison in Hypertensives, JNC 7 = Seventh Report of the Joint National Committee on Prevention, Detection, Evaluation, and Treatment of High Blood Pressure, UKPDS = United Kingdom Prospective Diabetes Study have favorable effects on glucose and lipid profiles, but as shown in ALLHAT, they are less efficacious on end points of stroke, heart failure, and overall CVD compared to thiazides.

References

1.   The Seventh Report of the Joint National Committee on Prevention, Detection, Evaluation, and Treatment of High Blood Pressure. JNC VII. US Department of Health and Human Services National Institutes of Health National Heart, Lung, and Blood Institute, National High Blood Pressure Education Program. NIH Publication No. 03-5233. May 2003.

2.   Anderson PJ, Critchley JA, Chan JC, et al: Factor analysis of the metabolic syndrome: obesity vs insulin resistance as the central abnormality. *Int J Obes Relat Metab Disord* 2001;25:1782-1788.

3.   Hanley AJ, Karter AJ, Festa A, et al: Factor analysis of metabolic syndrome using directly measured insulin sensitivity: The Insulin Resistance Atherosclerosis Study. *Diabetes* 2002;51:2642-2647.

4.   Kue Young T, Chateau D, Zhang M: Factor analysis of ethnic variation in the multiple metabolic (insulin resistance) syndrome in three Canadian populations. *Am J Human Biol* 2002;14:649-658.

5.   Hanson RL, Imperatore G, Bennett PH, et al: Components of the 'metabolic syndrome' and incidence of type 2 diabetes. *Diabetes* 2002;51:3120-3127.

6.   Howard BV, Criqui MH, Curb JD, et al: Risk factor clustering in the insulin resistance syndrome and its relationship to cardiovascular disease in postmenopausal white, black, hispanic, and Asian/Pacific Islander women. *Metabolism* 2003;52:362-371.

7.   Shen BJ, Todaro JF, Niaura R, et al: Are metabolic risk factors one unified syndrome? Modeling the structure of the metabolic syndrome X. *Am J Epidemiol* 2003;157:701-711.

8.   Ramachandran A, Snehalatha C, Satyavani K, et al: Metabolic syndrome in urban Asian Indian adults—a population study using modified ATP III criteria. *Diabetes Res Clin Pract* 2003;60:199-204.

9.   Novak S, Stapleton LM, Litaker JR, et al: A confirmatory factor analysis evaluation of the coronary heart disease risk factors of metabolic syndrome with emphasis on the insulin resistance factor. *Diabetes Obes Metab* 2003;5:388-396.

10. Hamann A, Sharma AM: Genetics of obesity and obesity-related hypertension. *Semin Nephrol* 2002;22:100-104.

11. Engeli S, Sharma AM: Emerging concepts in the pathophysiology and treatment of obesity-associated hypertension. *Curr Opin Cardiol* 2002;17:355-359.

12. Redon J: Hypertension in obesity. *Nutr Metab Cardiovasc Dis* 2001;11:344-353.

13. Montani JP, Antic V, Yang Z, et al: Pathways from obesity to hypertension: from the perspective of a vicious triangle. *Int J Obes Relat Metab Disord* 2002;26(suppl 2):S28-S38.

14. Rocchini AP: Insulin resistance, obesity and hypertension. *J Nutr* 1995;125(suppl 6):1718S-1724S.

15. Hall JE, Brands MW, Zappe DH, et al: Insulin resistance, hyperinsulinemia, and hypertension: causes, consequences, or merely correlations? *Proc Soc Exp Biol Med* 1995;208:317-329.

16. Berry C, Hamilton CA, Brosnan MJ, et al: Investigation into the sources of superoxide in human blood vessels: angiotensin II increases superoxide production in human internal mammary arteries. *Circulation* 2000;101:2206-2212.

17. Egan BM: Insulin resistance and the sympathetic nervous system. *Curr Hypertens Rep* 2003;5:247-254.

18. Schiffrin EL: A critical review of the role of endothelial factors in the pathogenesis of hypertension. *J Cardiovasc Pharmacol* 2001;38(suppl 2):S3-S6.

19. Black PH: The inflammatory response is an integral part of the stress response: Implications for atherosclerosis, insulin resistance, type II diabetes and metabolic syndrome X. *Brain Behav Immun* 2003;17:350-364.

20. Steinberg HO, Baron AD: Vascular function, insulin resistance and fatty acids. *Diabetologia* 2002;45:623-634. Epub 2002 Apr 2004.

21. Lewington S, Clarke R, Qizilbash N, et al: Age-specific relevance of usual blood pressure to vascular mortality: a meta-analysis of individual data for one million adults in 61 prospective studies. *Lancet* 2002;360:1903-1913.

22. Vasan RS, Beiser A, Seshadri S, et al: Residual lifetime risk for developing hypertension in middle-aged women and men: The Framingham Heart Study. *JAMA* 2002;287:1003-1010.

23. Neal B, MacMahon S, Chapman N: Effects of ACE inhibitors, calcium antagonists, and other blood-pressure-lowering drugs: Results of prospectively designed overviews of randomized trials. Blood Pressure Lowering Treatment Trialists' Collaboration. *Lancet* 2000;356:1955-1964.

24. Stamler J, Vaccaro O, Neaton JD, et al: Diabetes, other risk factors, and 12-yr cardiovascular mortality for men screened in the Multiple Risk Factor Intervention Trial. *Diabetes Care* 1993;16: 434-444.

25. Ogden LG, He J, Lydick E, et al: Long-term absolute benefit of lowering blood pressure in hypertensive patients according to the JNC VI risk stratification. *Hypertension* 2000;35:539-543.

26. Adler AI, Stratton IM, Neil HA, et al: Association of systolic blood pressure with macrovascular and microvascular complications of type 2 diabetes (UKPDS 36): prospective observational study. *BMJ* 2000;321:412-419.

27. Birkenhäger WH, Staessen JA, Gasowski J, et al: Effects of antihypertensive treatment on endpoints in the diabetic patients randomized in the Systolic Hypertension in Europe (Syst-Eur) trial. *J Nephrol* 2000;13:232-237.

28. Zanchetti A, Hansson L, Clement D, et al: Benefits and risks of more intensive blood pressure lowering in hypertensive patients of the HOT study with different risk profiles: does a J-shaped curve exist in smokers? *J Hypertens* 2003;21:797-804.

29. Effects of ramipril on cardiovascular and microvascular outcomes in people with diabetes mellitus: results of the HOPE study and MICRO-HOPE substudy. Heart Outcomes Prevention Evaluation Study Investigators. *Lancet* 2000;355:253-259.

30. Lewis EJ, Hunsicker LG, Bain RP, et al: The effect of angiotensin-converting-enzyme inhibition on diabetic nephropathy. The Collaborative Study Group. *N Engl J Med* 1993;329:1456-1462.

31. Maschio G, Alberti D, Janin G, et al: Effect of the angiotensin-converting-enzyme inhibitor benazepril on the progression of chronic renal insufficiency. The Angiotensin-Converting-Enzyme Inhibition in Progressive Renal Insufficiency Study Group. *N Engl J Med* 1996;334:939-945.

32. Ravid M, Lang R, Rachmani R, et al: Long-term renoprotective effect of angiotensin-converting enzyme inhibition in non-insulin-dependent diabetes mellitus. A 7-year follow-up study. *Arch Intern Med* 1996;156:286-289.

33. Dahlof B, Devereux RB, Kjeldsen SE, et al: Cardiovascular morbidity and mortality in the Losartan Intervention For Endpoint reduction in hypertension study (LIFE): a randomised trial against atenolol. *Lancet* 2002;359:995-1003.

34. Lindholm LH, Ibsen H, Dahlof B, et al: Cardiovascular morbidity and mortality in patients with diabetes in the Losartan Intervention For Endpoint reduction in hypertension study (LIFE): a randomised trial against atenolol. *Lancet* 2002;359:1004-1010.

35. Tatti P, Pahor M, Byington RP, et al: Outcome results of the Fosinopril Versus Amlodipine Cardiovascular Events Randomized Trial (FACET) in patients with hypertension and NIDDM. *Diabetes Care* 1998;21:597-603.

36. Estacio RO, Jeffers BW, Gifford N, et al: Effect of blood pressure control on diabetic microvascular complications in patients with hypertension and type 2 diabetes. *Diabetes Care* 2000;23(suppl 2):B54-B64.

37. Hansson L, Lindholm LH, Niskanen L, et al: Effect of angiotensin-converting-enzyme inhibition compared with conventional therapy on cardiovascular morbidity and mortality in hypertension: the Captopril Prevention Project (CAPPP) randomised trial. *Lancet* 1999;353:611-616.

38. Pahor M, Psaty BM, Alderman MH, et al: Therapeutic benefits of ACE inhibitors and other antihypertensive drugs in patients with type 2 diabetes. *Diabetes Care* 2000;23:888-892.

39. O'Connor CM, Carson PE, Miller AB, et al: Effect of amlodipine on mode of death among patients with advanced heart failure in the PRAISE trial. Prospective Randomized Amlodipine Survival Evaluation. *Am J Cardiol* 1998;82:881-887.

40. Sica DA, Douglas JG: The African American Study of Kidney Disease and Hypertension (AASK): new findings. *J Clin Hypertens* (Greenwich) 2001;3:244-251.

41. Moser M: Why are physicians not prescribing diuretics more frequently in the management of hypertension? *JAMA* 1998;279:1813-1816.

42. Zanella MT, Kohlmann O Jr, Ribeiro AB: Treatment of obesity hypertension and diabetes syndrome. *Hypertension* 2001;38 (3 pt 2):705-708.

43. Julius S, Majahalme S, Palatini P: Antihypertensive treatment of patients with diabetes and hypertension. *Am J Hypertens* 2001; 14(11 pt 2):310S-316S.

44. Imazu M: Hypertension and insulin disorders. *Curr Hypertens Rep* 2002;4:477-482.

45. Tourniaire J, Bajard L, Harfouch M, et al: [Restoration of insulin sensitivity after correction of hypokalemia due to chronic tubulopathy in a diabetic patient] *Diabete Metab* 1988;14:717-720. [Article in French]

46. Wing LM, Reid CM, Ryan P, et al: A comparison of outcomes with angiotensin converting-enzyme inhibitors and diuretics for hypertension in the elderly. *N Engl J Med* 2003;348:583-592.

47. Psaty BM, Lumley T, Furberg CD, et al: Health outcomes associated with various antihypertensive therapies used as first-line agents: a network meta-analysis. *JAMA* 2003;289:2534-2544.

48. Nosadini R, Tonolo G: Relationship between blood glucose control, pathogenesis and progression of diabetic nephropathy. *J Am Soc Nephrol* 2004;15(suppl 1):S1-S5.

49. Punzi HA, Punzi CF: Metabolic issues in the antihypertensive and lipid-lowering heart attack trial study. *Curr Hypertens Rep* 2004;6:106-110.

50. Pitt B, Zannad F, Remme WJ, et al: The effect of spironolactone on morbidity and mortality in patients with severe heart failure. Randomized Aldactone Evaluation Study Investigators. *N Engl J Med* 1999;341:709-717.

51. Effectiveness of spironolactone added to an angiotensin-converting enzyme inhibitor and a loop diuretic for severe chronic congestive heart failure (the Randomized Aldactone Evaluation Study [RALES]). *Am J Cardiol* 1996;78:902-907.

52. Soberman JE, Weber KT: Spironolactone in congestive heart failure. *Curr Hypertens Rep* 2000;2:451-456.

53. Pitt B, Williams G, Remme W, et al: The EPHESUS trial: eplerenone in patients with heart failure due to systolic dysfunction complicating acute myocardial infarction. Eplerenone Post-AMI Heart Failure Efficacy and Survival Study. *Cardiovasc Drugs Ther* 2001;15:79-87.

54. Brenner BM, Cooper ME, de Zeeuw D, et al: Effects of losartan on renal and cardiovascular outcomes in patients with type 2 diabetes and nephropathy. *N Engl J Med* 2001;345:861-869.

55. Lewis EJ, Hunsicker LG, Clarke WR, et al: Renoprotective effect of the angiotensin-receptor antagonist irbesartan in patients with nephropathy due to type 2 diabetes. *N Engl J Med* 2001;345:851-860.

56. Gerth WC, Remuzzi G, Viberti G, et al: Losartan reduces the burden and cost of ESRD: public health implications from the RENAAL study for the European Union. *Kidney Int* 2002;62 (suppl 82):68-72.

57. Garg R, Yusuf S: Overview of randomized trials of angiotensin-converting enzyme inhibitors on mortality and morbidity in patients with heart failure. Collaborative Group on ACE Inhibitor Trials. *JAMA* 1995;273:1450-1456.

58. Sowers JR: SUNY School of Medicine. Personal communication.

59. Schiffrin EL, Canadian Institutes of Health Research Multidisciplinary Research Group on Hypertension: Beyond blood pressure: the endothelium and atherosclerosis progression. *Am J Hypertens* 2002;15(10 pt 2):115S-122S.

60. Ma LJ, Nakamura S, Whitsitt JS, et al: Regression of sclerosis in aging by an angiotensin inhibition-induced decrease in PAI-1. *Kidney Int* 2000;58:2425-2436.

61. Cohn JN, Tognoni G, Valsartan Heart Failure Trial Investigators: A randomized trial of the angiotensin-receptor blocker valsartan in chronic heart failure. *N Engl J Med* 2001;345:1667-1675.

62. Struckman DR, Rivey MP: Combined therapy with an angiotensin II receptor blocker and an angiotensin-converting enzyme inhibitor in heart failure. *Ann Pharmacother* 2001;35:242-248.

63. Cohn JN: Interaction of beta-blockers and angiotensin receptor blockers/ACE inhibitors in heart failure. *J Renin Angiotensin Aldosterone Syst* 2003;4:137-139.

64. Dimopoulos K, Salukhe TV, Coats AJ, et al: Meta-analyses of mortality and morbidity effects of an angiotensin receptor blocker in patients with chronic heart failure already receiving an ACE inhibitor (alone or with a beta-blocker). *Int J Cardiol* 2004;93:105-111.

65. Padwal R, Laupacis A: Antihypertensive therapy and incidence of type 2 diabetes: a systematic review. *Diabetes Care* 2004;27:247-255.

66. Brook RD: Mechanism of differential effects of antihypertensive agents on serum lipids. *Curr Hypertens Rep* 2000;2:370-377.

67. ALLHAT Collaborative Research Group: Major cardiovascular events in hypertensive patients randomized to doxazosin vs chlorthalidone: the antihypertensive and lipid-lowering treatment to prevent heart attack trial (ALLHAT). *JAMA* 2000;283:1967-1975.

68. Landsberg L, Young JB: Physiology and pharmacology of the autonomic nervous system. In: *Harrison's Principles of Internal Medicine*, 14th ed. Isselbacher K et al, eds. New York, McGraw-Hill, 1998.

69. Foster DW, Rubenstein AH: Hypoglycemia. In: *Harrison's Principles of Internal Medicine*, 14th ed. Isselbacher K et al, eds. New York, McGraw-Hill, 1998.

70. Tight blood pressure control and risk of macrovascular and microvascular complications in type 2 diabetes: UKPDS 38. UK Prospective Diabetes Study Group. *BMJ* 1998;317:703-713.

71. Bakris GL, Fonseca V, Katholi RE, et al: Metabolic effects of carvedilol vs metoprolol in patients with type 2 diabetes mellitus and hypertension: a randomized controlled trial. *JAMA* 2004;292:2227-2236.

72. The ALLHAT Officers and Coordinators for the ALLHAT Collaborative Research Group: The Antihypertensive and Lipid-Lowering Treatment to Prevent Heart Attack Trial (ALLHAT). Major outcomes in high-risk hypertensive patients randomized to angiotensinconverting enzyme inhibitor or calcium channel blocker vs diuretic: The Antihypertensive and Lipid-Lowering Treatment to Prevent Heart Attack Trial (ALLHAT). *JAMA* 2002;288:2981-2997.

73. Williams GH: Hypertensive vascular disease. In: *Harrison's Principles of Internal Medicine*, 14th ed. Isselbacher K et al, eds. New York, McGraw-Hill, 1998.

74. Drug Facts and Comparisons. St Louis, 2000.

75. Jukema JW, van der Hoorn JW: Amlodipine and atorvastatin in atherosclerosis: a review of the potential of combination therapy. *Expert Opin Pharmacother* 2004;5:459-468.

76. Jukema JW, Zwinderman AH, van Boven AJ, et al: Evidence for a synergistic effect of calcium channel blockers with lipid-lowering therapy in retarding progression of coronary atherosclerosis in symptomatic patients with normal to moderately raised cholesterol levels. The REGRESS Study Group. *Arterioscler Thromb Vasc Biol* 1996;16:425-430.

77. Liebovitz E, Beniashvili M, Zimlichmn R, et al: Treatment with amlodipine and atorvastatin has additive effect in improvement of arterial compliance in hypertensive hyperlipidemic patients. *Am J Hypertens* 2003;(9 pt 1):715-718.

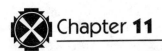 Chapter **11**

The Metabolic Syndrome: Summary Recommendations

The metabolic syndrome represents a clustering of risk factors for atherosclerotic cardiovascular disease (ASCVD).[1] Nearly 25% of the adult population in the United States is now estimated to have the metabolic syndrome.[2] Although ASCVD must be considered the most important clinical end point in the United States, the association between the metabolic syndrome and type 2 diabetes is strong,[3] and even prominent in many countries.

Pathogenesis of the Metabolic Syndrome

The two dominant underlying risk factors of the metabolic syndrome are obesity and insulin resistance.[3] Obese adipose tissue is increasingly being recognized as the producer of factors that contribute to the development of the metabolic syndrome, including excess nonesterified fatty acids, cytokines (tumor necrosis factor-α [TNF-α]), resistin, adiponectin, leptin, and plasminogen activator inhibitor-1 (PAI-1). A notable feature of the metabolic syndrome is accumulation of fat in tissue outside of adipose tissue, notably, muscle and liver. This ectopic deposition of fat appears to play an important role in development of metabolic risk factors. Beyond obesity, other abnormalities of adipose tissue are associated with the metabolic syndrome, including abdominal obesity[4] and lipodystrophy.[5]

Most people with the metabolic syndrome display some degree of insulin resistance, which many investigators[6,7] regard as the clinical heart of the metabolic syndrome. Clearly, insulin resistance is a major underlying risk factor for type 2 diabetes. Although insulin resistance is strongly associated with metabolic risk factors for ASCVD, evidence that it is a direct cause is less clear. Various plausible mechanisms have been proposed to explain how insulin resistance could induce these risk factors.[6,7] Perhaps the best opportunity for understanding the relation between insulin resistance and metabolic risk factors lies in further study of cases of primary (genetic) insulin resistance.[8] Preliminary evidence suggests that genetic forms of insulin resistance may produce mild aberrations in metabolic risk factors independent of obesity. Moreover, in some persons, obesity and primary insulin resistance may together exacerbate these risk factors.

Other underlying risk factors for the metabolic syndrome include physical inactivity, aging, atherogenic diets, and hormonal imbalance.[3] Physical inactivity worsens insulin resistance and promotes development of obesity. Loss of muscle mass and increase in body fat commonly accompany aging. Aging muscle further exhibits some loss in ability to oxidize fatty acids, which will increase insulin resistance. Postulated endocrine abnormalities underlying the metabolic syndrome include polycystic ovary disease and mild hypercorticoidism as causes of abdominal obesity.

Genetic heterogeneity affects expression of lipoprotein metabolism, blood pressure levels, insulin secretory capacity, coagulation and fibrinolysis factors, and inflammatory responses. Thus, the genetic architecture for each of these systems falls under the influence of the underlying risk factors.

Table 11-1: Diagnosing the Metabolic Syndrome*

Factor	Defining Level
Abdominal obesity	Waist circumference
-Men	≥102 cm (≥40 in)
-Women	≥88 cm (≥35 in)
Triglycerides	≥150 mg/dL
HDL cholesterol	
-Men	<40 mg/dL
-Women	<50 mg/dL
Blood pressure	≥130 mm Hg systolic or ≥85 mm Hg diastolic
Fasting glucose	≥100 mg/dL

*From NCEP ATP III guidelines.

Clinical Diagnosis of the Metabolic Syndrome

For many years the metabolic syndrome was more of a concept than a clinical entity. In recent years, several groups have formulated clinical criteria for the diagnosis of the metabolic syndrome. Among these are the World Health Organization (WHO),[9] the United States National Cholesterol Education Program (NCEP) Adult Treatment Panel III (ATP III),[1] and the American Association of Clinical Endocrinologists (AACE).[10] The ATP III criteria represent an evolutionary stage developed from WHO criteria. They emphasize abdominal obesity as the major underlying risk factor for the metabolic syndrome. They contrast with the WHO criteria, which place primary emphasis on insulin resistance. AACE likewise emphasizes insulin resistance as the driving force of the syndrome and prefers to call it the *insulin resistance syndrome*. ATP III criteria have the advantage over WHO and AACE criteria in their simplicity, convenience, and lower cost. According to ATP III, a diagnosis of the metabolic syndrome can be made when a patient has three of the five characteristics listed in Table 11-1.

Other components not routinely measured are reported to be common in persons with insulin resistance and the metabolic syndrome. These include elevated apolipoprotein B (apo B), small low-density lipoprotein (LDL) particles, insulin resistance and hyperinsulinemia, impaired glucose tolerance, elevated C-reactive protein (CRP), and coagulation factors (eg, PAI-1 and fibrinogen). Although apo B levels often are elevated, LDL-cholesterol levels may not be increased. Their measurement in clinical practice is optional, and we do not now know how their detection will modify clinical management of patients with ATP III criteria for the metabolic syndrome.

Risk Assessment in Patients With the Metabolic Syndrome

A commonly asked question is whether the metabolic syndrome itself can be used to assess the likelihood of developing ASCVD. Prospective studies[11] have shown that individuals with the metabolic syndrome are at increased risk for ASCVD. Recently, investigators of the Framingham Heart Study carried out an analysis to determine the absolute risk for ASCVD associated with the metabolic syndrome.[3] It seems evident that a condition characterized by multiple risk factors will carry a greater risk for adverse clinical outcomes than will a single risk factor. This conclusion is implicit in Framingham risk equations, which incorporate many of the components of the metabolic syndrome. The Framingham analysis was based on Framingham study offspring (men and women, mean age 52 years) who were followed for 8 years. The investigators found that the metabolic syndrome alone predicted approximately 25% of all new-onset ASCVD. This percentage was largely unaffected by whether diabetes was included in the metabolic syndrome criteria. In the absence of diabetes, people with the metabolic syndrome rarely exhibited a 10-year risk for CHD exceeding 20%, which is designated high-risk by ATP III. Most men with the metabolic syndrome had a 10-year risk of 10% to 20%, which ATP III calls moderately high risk. Framingham women with the metabolic syndrome usually had lower risk (ie, a 10-year risk for major coronary events less than 10%). Importantly, Framingham investigators showed that a diagnosis of the metabolic syndrome provides a less-accurate assessment of 10-year risk than does the Framingham risk scoring procedure that makes use of all of the major risk factors. Thus, the metabolic syndrome per se should not be used for global risk assessment. Instead, standard risk algorithms are preferred for this purpose.[1]

The Metabolic Syndrome as a Predictor of Diabetes

According to Framingham investigators, the metabolic syndrome is highly predictive of new-onset diabetes.[3] The relative risk for developing type 2 diabetes is approximately five-fold higher in persons with the metabolic syndrome than in those without it. The predictive power for diabetes may be enhanced by carrying out an oral glucose tolerance test. An oral glucose tolerance test (OGTT) may identify patients who are normoglycemic but have impaired glucose tolerance. These patients will likely be at higher risk for developing type 2 diabetes than those who remain glucose tolerant.

Management of Underlying Risk Factors

First-line therapy of the metabolic syndrome is to modify the underlying risk factors: overweight and obesity, physical inactivity, and an atherogenic diet. Clinical management represents an extension of the public health approach to risk reduction. When a person is identified by ATP III criteria to have the metabolic syndrome, he or she should enter clinical management. The physician should set the goals of treatment, encourage lifestyle modification, and involve additional health professionals as necessary.

Overweight and Obesity

Treatment of obesity should follow the guidelines developed by the National Institutes of Health in 1998.[12] According to these guidelines,[12] overweight and obesity are defined as body mass indexes (BMIs) of 25 to 29.9 kg/m^2 and ≥30 kg/m^2, respectively. Abdominal obesity was added to the classification and was defined as a waist circumference ≥102 cm (≥40 inches) in men and ≥88 cm (≥35 inches) in women. Abdominal obesity appears to be strongly associated with the metabolic risk factors for ASCVD.[12] ATP III recommends that abdominal obesity be one of the clinical criteria for diagnosis of the metabolic syndrome. However, some persons will manifest the metabolic syndrome at waist circumferences less than the categoric cut points listed in the obesity guidelines.

Weight reduction in obese persons will help to reverse most of the metabolic risk factors.[12] The essential approach to weight reduction involves behavior changes to reduce caloric intake and increase physical activity. Treatment guidelines emphasize certain key points. For example, 'crash diets' and 'extreme diets' rarely achieve long-term weight reduction. More effective for long-term weight loss is moderate reduction in caloric intake that eliminates about 500 to 1,000 calories a day. A realistic goal for weight reduction is 7% to 10% over the first 6 to 12 months. To achieve long-term weight loss, addition of regular physical activity is usually required. A key point for long-term success is the need for behavior modification. Dieting alone is rarely successful. Behavior modification includes an improvement in eating habits. Among the habits that typically cause weight gain are a failure to plan meals ahead of time, failure to choose lower-calorie foods (eg, failure to read labels), snacking between meals and at bedtime, overeating at meals (eg, large portions, second helpings, desserts), frequent dining out, and being prone to eating binges. Useful techniques of

**Table 11-2: Key Features of
Dietary Recommendations**

- **Choose a variety of fruits and vegetables daily**
- **Avoid excess dietary saturated fat**
  - Choose a diet that is low in saturated fat
    and cholesterol and moderate in total fat
  - Replace saturated fats with unsaturated oils
- **Avoid excess dietary carbohydrates**
  - For carbohydrates, emphasize grain foods,
    especially whole grains
  - Choose beverages and foods to moderate intake
    of sugars
- **Choose and prepare foods with less salt**
- **If you drink alcoholic beverages, do so
  in moderation**

Modified from Dietary Guidelines for Americans, US
Departments of Agriculture and Health and Human
Services, 2000.

behavior modification include family support, managing and
preventing periods of stress, and daily exercise. For moti-
vated patients, the obesity guidelines for weight reduction
can be obtained online at www.nhlbi.nih.gov and
www.americanheart.org. An understanding of principles of
behavior modification is important but frequently insufficient. For many patients in clinical management, professional
support (eg, nutritional counseling) can assist in achieving
weight reduction.

Physical Inactivity

Most American adults are sedentary. This is unfortu-
nate because regular physical activity promotes weight
reduction, reduces insulin resistance, mitigates metabolic

risk factors, and reduces risk for several chronic diseases. Among the latter are ASCVD and type 2 diabetes. Physical inactivity is an underlying risk factor for the metabolic syndrome. The American Heart Association (AHA) provides physical activity guidelines that are moderate and practical.[13] The basic recommendation is a daily minimum of 30 minutes of moderate-intensity physical activity. Some additional benefit is achieved by increasing exercise time to 1 hour a day. Suggestions that may promote increased physical activity include:[14]

- Walking briskly (10 to 15 minutes) several times per day
- Adding exercise to daily habits (brisk walking, jogging, swimming, biking, golfing, team sports)
- Substituting exercise activities for television viewing and computer games
- Purchasing simple exercise equipment for the home (eg, treadmill).

Dietary Modification

The Dietary Guidelines for Americans, set forth by the US Departments of Agriculture and Health and Human Services, offer a reasonable dietary approach for managing patients with the metabolic syndrome.[15] The key features of dietary recommendations based on these guidelines and those of the ATP III panel are listed in Table 11-2.

The AHA (www.americanheart.org) provides useful information on how to choose a healthy eating pattern that will reduce risk for ASCVD in patients with the metabolic syndrome.

Management of Individual Metabolic Risk Factors

Atherogenic Dyslipidemia

In patients with the metabolic syndrome who have atherogenic dyslipidemia, the primary target of therapy is elevated apo B-containing lipoproteins. The best indicators for these lipoproteins are LDL plus very low-density lipoprotein cholesterol (VLDL-C) (non-high-density lipoprotein cholesterol [non-HDL-C]) or total apo B.[1] For high-risk patients (10-year risk for major coronary events >20%), the goal of therapy is to reduce LDL + VLDL-C to <130 mg/dL (or apo B to <90 mg/dL). For those at moderately high risk (10-year risk 10% to 20%), the goal of therapy is LDL + VLDL-C <160 mg/dL (or apo B <120 mg/dL). For both categories of risk, statin therapy usually is indicated. Statins reduce both LDL-apo B and VLDL-apo B. In many patients, the goal can be achieved with statin therapy alone.

If triglyceride levels remain elevated after statin therapy in patients at high or moderately high risk, physicians should consider adding a fibrate or nicotinic acid.[1] The preferred fibrate to use in combination with a statin is fenofibrate (TriCor®, Lofibra™) because the combination of a statin and gemfibrozil (Lopid®) carries too high a risk for severe myopathy. Available data indicate that the combination of a statin and fenofibrate carries a lower risk for myopathy. When fenofibrate is used in combination with a statin, there often is some additional lowering of total apo B (or LDL + VLDL-C), but the combination offers three advantages. First, fenofibrate reduces atherogenic remnant lipoproteins; second, it transforms smaller LDL to larger LDL; and third, it raises HDL-C more than statins alone.[16] The same benefits are achieved by combining a statin with nicotinic acid. Unfortunately, nicotinic acid often causes bothersome side effects, including flushing and itching of the skin, gastrointestinal distress, rises in plasma glucose and uric acid, and abnormal liver function tests. Both flushing and abnormal liver function tests can be minimized by use of an extended-release niacin preparation (Niaspan®). Long-acting preparations carry too high a risk for liver dysfunction, while crystalline nicotinic acid more often causes severe flushing. When nicotinic acid is used with statin therapy, the dose should be kept relatively low (1 to 2 g/d).

When patients with the metabolic syndrome and atherogenic dyslipidemia have a 10-year risk <10% (lower to moderate risk), drug therapy should be used only when the LDL + VLDL-C (or apo B) is high (ie, LDL + VLDL-C >190 mg/dL or apo B >140 mg/dL). Otherwise, lifestyle therapies should be emphasized.

Elevated Blood Pressure

The Seventh Report of the Joint National Committee on Prevention, Detection, Evaluation, and Treatment of High Blood Pressure (JNC 7)[17] recommends the use of antihypertensive drugs when blood pressure exceeds 140 mm Hg systolic or 90 mm Hg diastolic on repeated measurements. The primary goal of therapy is to reduce blood pressure to <140/90 mm Hg. In patients with established diabetes, JNC 7 sets a lower goal, <130/80 mm Hg. JNC 7 did not identify particular antihypertensive agents as preferable for hypertensive patients with the metabolic syndrome. However, thiazide diuretics and β-blockers in high doses can accentuate insulin resistance and worsen atherogenic dyslipidemia. In the metabolic syndrome, higher doses of thiazides can cause an elevation of glucose to categoric diabetes in patients with impaired glucose tolerance. Therefore, doses of thiazide diuretics should be relatively low. Despite a worsening of glucose tolerance, β-blockers protect against sudden death in patients with established ASCVD; consequently, they are not contraindicated in patients with type 2 diabetes and ASCVD. Angiotensin-converting enzyme (ACE) inhibitors and angiotensin-receptor blockers (ARBs) are especially attractive for patients with the metabolic syndrome because they are renoprotective and have been shown to reduce risk for new-onset ASCVD. Several clinical trials, but not all, point to advantages of ACE inhibitors and ARBs over other drugs in patients with diabetes.[17]

Insulin Resistance and Hyperglycemia

A fundamental question is whether drug treatment of insulin resistance will reduce the risk for developing type 2 diabetes and, if so, whether it is cost-effective. Evidence is growing that drugs can reduce risk for conversion of impaired glucose tolerance into categorical hyperglycemia (or diabetes). Metformin (Glucophage®) therapy in patients with prediabetes reduced the risk for conversion to diabetes.[18]

Insulin resistance is associated with increased ASCVD risk. In one clinical trial, metformin therapy appeared to decrease the risk for new-onset ASCVD in an obese subgroup.[19] Further studies with metformin are required to document a cardioprotective effect. None of the glitazones (thiazolidinediones) has been documented to reduce risk for ASCVD, but these agents are being tested in clinical trials.

These considerations lead to the issue of how best to treat insulin resistance and hyperglycemia in patients with type 2 diabetes. When hyperglycemia develops in patients with the metabolic syndrome, the risk for ASCVD rises. In patients with type 2 diabetes, priority must be given to appropriate treatment of dyslipidemia and hypertension. Drug therapy of each has been documented to reduce risk for ASCVD.[1,17] A strong case can be made for improved glycemic control as well. Most importantly, good glycemic control will reduce risk for microvascular disease and other diabetic complications. For these reasons, a reduction in glycated hemoglobin (Hb A_{1c}) level to <7.0% is indicated. Whether better control will reduce ASCVD events remains to be documented in controlled clinical trials, although circumstantial evidence strongly suggests that it will.

Prothrombotic State

The various prothrombotic factors typical of the metabolic syndrome, including elevations of fibrinogen and PAI-1, are not routinely measured in clinical practice. Nonetheless, in both primary and secondary prevention, thrombotic events can be reduced by aspirin therapy. The AHA has recommended use of low-dose aspirin (81 mg/d) for most patients whose 10-year risk for CHD is >10%, as determined by Framingham risk scoring.[20] When patients with the metabolic syndrome have a 10-year risk for major coronary events >10%, aspirin prophylaxis should be considered.

Proinflammatory State

This condition is best recognized by elevations of CRP, but various inflammatory cytokines (eg, TNF-α, IL-6) and fibrinogen are commonly elevated as well. Patients with the metabolic syndrome typically have elevations in CRP levels (eg, >3 mg/dL).[21] There is no specific therapy for high levels of CRP. Nonetheless, weight reduction and many of the drugs used to treat metabolic risk factors will lower CRP. This change could represent a dampening of the proinflammatory state.

References

1. Third Report of the National Cholesterol Education Program (NCEP) Expert Panel on Detection, Evaluation, and Treatment of High Blood Cholesterol in Adults (Adult Treatment Panel III) final report. *Circulation* 2002;106:3143-3421.

2. Ford ES, Giles WH, Dietz WH: Prevalence of the metabolic syndrome among US adults: findings from the third National Health and Nutrition Survey. *JAMA* 2002;287:356-359.

3. Grundy SM, Brewer HB Jr, Cleeman JI, et al: Definition of metabolic syndrome: report of the National Heart, Lung, and Blood Institute/American Heart Association conference on scientific issues related to definition. *Circulation* 2004;109:433-438.

4. Frayn KN: Visceral fat and insulin resistance—causative or correlative? *Br J Nutr* 2000;83(suppl 1):S71-S77.

5. Garg A: Acquired and inherited lipodystrophies. *N Engl J Med* 2004;350:1220-1234.

6. Reaven GM: Banting lecture 1988. Role of insulin resistance in human disease. *Diabetes* 1988;37:1595-1607.

7. Ferrannini E, Haffner SM, Mitchell BD: Hyperinsulinemia: the key feature of a cardiovascular and metabolic syndrome. *Diabetologia* 1991;34:416-422.

8. Abate N, Carulli L, Cabo-Chan A Jr, et al: Genetic polymorphism PC-1 K121Q and ethnic susceptibility to insulin resistance. *Clin Endocrinol Metab* 2003;88:5927-5934.

9.   Alberti KG, Zimmet PZ: Definition, diagnosis and classification of diabetes mellitus and its complications. Part 1: diagnosis and classification of diabetes mellitus provisional report of a WHO consultation. *Diabet Med* 1998;15:539-553.

10.   Einhorn D, Reaven GM, Cobin RH, et al: American College of Endocrinology position statement on insulin resistance syndrome. *Endocr Pract* 2003;9:237-252.

11.   Lakka HM, Laaksonen DE, Lakka TA, et al: The metabolic syndrome and total and cardiovascular disease mortality in middle-aged men. *JAMA* 2002;288:2709-2716.

12.   Clinical Guidelines on the Identification, Evaluation, and Treatment of Overweight and Obesity in Adults—The Evidence Report. National Institutes of Health. *Obes Res* 1998;6(suppl 2):51S-209S.

13.   Thompson PD, Buchner D, Pina IL, et al: Exercise and physical activity in the prevention and treatment of atherosclerotic cardiovascular disease: a statement from the Council on Clinical Cardiology (Subcommittee on Exercise, Rehabilitation, and Prevention) and the Council on Nutrition, Physical Activity, and Metabolism (Subcommittee on Physical Activity). *Circulation* 2003;107:3109-3116.

14.   Grundy SM, Hansen B, Smith SC Jr, et al: Clinical management of metabolic syndrome: report of the American Heart Association/National Heart, Lung, and Blood Institute/American Diabetes Association conference on scientific issues related to management. *Circulation* 2004;109:551-556.

15.   US Department of Agriculture and US Department of Health and Human Services. Nutrition and your health: dietary guidelines for Americans, 5th ed. Home and Garden Bulletin no. 232. Washington, DC, US Department of Agriculture, 2000, 44 pages.

16.   Vega GL, Ma PT, Cater NB, et al: Effects of adding fenofibrate (200 mg/d) to simvastatin (10 mg/d) in patients with combined hyperlipidemia and metabolic syndrome. *Am J Cardiol* 2003; 91:956-960.

17.   Chobanian AV, Bakris GL, Black HR, et al: The Seventh Report of the Joint National Committee on Prevention, Detection, Evaluation, and Treatment of High Blood Pressure: the JNC 7 report. *JAMA* 2003;289:2560-2572.

18.   Knowler WC, Barrett-Connor E, Fowler SE, et al: Reduction in the incidence of type 2 diabetes with lifestyle intervention or metformin. *N Engl J Med* 2002;346:393-403.

19. UK Prospective Diabetes Study (UKPDS) Group: Effect of intensive blood-glucose control with metformin on complications in overweight patients with type 2 diabetes. *Lancet* 1998;352:854-865.

20. Pearson TA, Blair SN, Daniels SR, et al: AHA Guidelines for Primary Prevention of Cardiovascular Disease and Stroke: 2002 Update: Consensus Panel Guide to Comprehensive Risk Reduction for Adult Patients Without Coronary or Other Atherosclerotic Vascular Diseases. American Heart Association Science Advisory and Coordinating Committee. *Circulation* 2002;106:388-391.

21. Ridker PM, Buring JE, Cook NR, et al: C-reactive protein, the metabolic syndrome, and risk of incident cardiovascular events: an 8-year follow-up of 14,719 initially healthy American women. *Circulation* 2003;107:391-397.

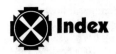 **Index**